BODY, MIND & SPIRIT

BODY, MIND & SPIRIT

The Journey Toward Health and Wholeness

EDITED BY Peter Albright, M.D. &
Bets Parker Albright

THE STEPHEN GREENE PRESS
Brattleboro, Vermont

This book is for all of you, everywhere, who seek for yourselves and for others the beautiful balance that is vibrant health. We dedicate it with love to the children of the world, with special thoughts directed toward our own; and to our fellow writers, whose energies came together to create the wholeness of the book.

This book has been produced in the United States of America. It is designed by IRVING PERKINS ASSOCIATES, and published by THE STEPHEN GREENE PRESS, Brattleboro, Vermont 05301.

Library of Congress Cataloging in Publication Data
Main entry under title:

Body, mind & spirit.

Bibliography: p.
Includes index.
1. Health. 2. Mind and body. 3. Holistic medicine. I. Albright, Peter, 1926– II. Albright, Elizabeth, 1920–
RA776.5.B63   613   80–12671
ISBN 0–8289–0385–9

Contents

ACKNOWLEDGMENTS

This book would never have happened without the energetic initiative and the ever-present support and encouragement of Bill Eastman, "our man from Stephen Greene." We also want to acknowledge that the quality of what developed was influenced by the work of Orion Barber, Castle Freeman, and the staff of The Stephen Greene Press. We have also been given valuable assistance by Caroline Otis and Bernie Flynn of Northern Lights Bookshop in St. Johnsbury, Vermont, for which we are very grateful.

Introduction

This is a book about *holism*, as it was originally described and as it has evolved to the present time. The first use of the word *holism* was in the 1926 book *Holism and Evolution* by Jan Christiaan Smuts, the famous South African soldier-statesman-philosopher. He coined the term *holism* (from ολος = whole) to mean a "fundamental factor operative towards the creation of wholes in the universe."[1]

General Smuts stated that wholes are not mere artificial constructions of thought, but are something real in the universe. He said that "The idea of wholes and wholeness should therefore not be confined to the biological domain; it covers both inorganic substances and the highest manifestations of the human spirit. Taking a plant or an animal as a type of a whole, we notice the fundamental holistic characters as a unity of parts which is so close and intense as to be more than the sum of its parts."[2]

In the 1980's the words *holism* and *holistic* are being tossed about as enthusiastically as a frisbee in the springtime. Countless articles in newspapers and magazines, and many books which deal with this "new" movement, are appearing on bookstore shelves. The reader and the listener can quickly become confused when an idea that contains the word *whole* appears to be broken down into such a vast number of separate techniques and approaches. Unless we are very clear about holism, we are in danger of falling into the same traps that snare us in our present super-specialized world!

In our view, holism and holistic health essentially involve the unity of body, mind, and spirit. A sound mind in a sound body— of course, we aim at that. We can and must study the body and mind together. It is more difficult to "study" the spirit, but, unless we find ways to become better acquainted with the spirit and aware of its vital involvement with the mind and body, our search for a new model for the New Age will be a vain one.

This book presents a framework to help orient your thinking

toward a cohesive concept of health, healing, and wholeness. In the first section is a vision, a vision of ourselves, really, with all aspects of our humanness considered, not just physical or mental sickness or health. We then invite you to look at the essential nature of the healing process as it can presently be understood. You are exhorted to take charge of your own life, and, at the same time, to learn when outside help is needed.

The second section shows us the world of sickness and health as we know it, briefly scanning the many centuries of health history leading up to the present. The inability of the scientific-medical model to deal with all aspects of human health is discussed. Various by-products of this model, such as the powerful drug and technological industries and vast multi-media programming for sickness, are described in some detail. An historical account of how cancer has been viewed over the past few decades will illustrate a number of the points made in this section. Finally, we look at our stirrings and stretchings over the past few years, which have led to the larger holistic concepts of health and wholeness. We watch man begin to move toward a new range of possibilities for life on this planet.

The third and fourth sections draw attention, in turn, to a number of individual areas of concern about health, describing how newer concepts and strategies are developing in each area. The various stages of human development, from conception through death and beyond, are studied. The role of optimal nourishment for the entire organism is stressed. The importance of shaping our attitudes, working with our bodies, and getting acquainted with our spirit in a thoroughly integrated way is discussed at some length. Then we return to a more focused consideration of the healing process in several specific aspects. A special consideration of the physics of energy in human biology and its involvement in healing is of particular interest in understanding some scientifically measurable aspects of healing energy. The section concludes with some projections and speculations on the role of orthodox medicine in the holistic era.

The final section brings us back to look at our original picture of health and wholeness, to see if what we have been describing will really help individuals progress toward realizing vibrant health. In particular, we want to examine the concept of the holistic health center. Then we consider the future of health care generally, that is, what our best thoughts and plans are about how our vision can be made real for the millions of people in the world, whether it be through some great system of organization, or the development of therapeutic communities, or by a combination of many methods. The section and the book close with the realization that the best solution for our civilization will come through the efforts of a vast network of loving and caring people working together to heal the planet.

In organizing this book, we have given very careful thought to the people who would contribute to its wholeness and uniqueness. We have been wonderfully fortunate both in meeting exciting, gifted and loving people in our travels, and in knowing, and sometimes being related to, equally exciting people nearby.

The people who are writing about techniques and approaches to holistic health in this book are not presenting their pitch as the total answer. They are thoughtful, wise, and dedicated folk who have found that they resonate especially well to a certain approach. They have studied and mastered their art and offer it as a valid means of improving health, not as the whole answer.

If we are not very clear about why we are presenting this book to you, your inevitable reaction will be: I wonder why they included some techniques and approaches and left others out! Certainly there *are* others, whom we do not know, who could have made similarly beautiful contributions. We are forced to choose a limited number in order to keep this book fairly short and readable.

As you read the chapters, we believe and hope that you will find, as we have, the unity flowing through all of them. There is a variety of ideas, techniques, and philosophies, but there are no basic contradictions. It all *works*. You, our readers, have the task of putting together for yourselves the pieces that fit best for you.

We hope that you will be excited, stimulated, and challenged to continue reading beyond the covers of this book. We hope that you will discover new chapters for yourselves and new friends in the realm of holism. We hope in time to know many of you!

We hope that you will feel that we have given you a well-balanced "meal," and that you realize, as we do, that there are many other menus that would contribute as well to the nourishment of your total needs.

This book is not simply a collection of articles about different subjects. It should not be read as a list of ways to achieve whole-ness. We think of it as a group of loving people holding hands in a circle and allowing the energy to flow. All of you are welcome into the circle. We stretch our hands out to you and enlarge the circle!

BETS AND PETER ALBRIGHT

PART I
Health and Wholeness: A Vision of Well-Being

1

The Triune Concept

PAUL SOLOMON

There was a time when all healers were priests and all priests were teachers. It may seem archaic to turn to a religious leader for treatment of the body, or to think that an educator is concerned with physical health or spiritual well-being. Yet that is the holistic principle. Man is a triune being. He thinks of himself as body, mind and spirit.

In our age of specialization, man has entrusted his "three selves" to specialists. He wouldn't think of asking his physician for spiritual advice, or his educator for treatment of physical disorders. Somewhere in our past, we decided to separate these three selves and pretend that one has no effect upon the others.

Perhaps this separation was a matter of convenience or expedience. Surely a seminarian has enough to study just to prepare for taking responsibility for man's relationship with God. Surely the physician has enough responsibility keeping the body mechanics running smoothly, and the educator finds enough challenge in teaching people how to learn and what to learn. In fact, the division seems so neat and the complexity of the interfaces so overwhelming that we might even be tempted to leave well enough alone. The physician has more than enough to do researching chemical complexities and bioenergies we don't yet understand. How can he possibly add to his physiological frontier additional considerations of spiritual welfare and psychological belief structures? The psychologist and the minister seem equally overwhelmed with the challenges of their respective disciplines.

This need to dissect and examine each separate component of human life may have originally led to specialization. The specialization, of course, has become increasingly specific, so that today we find the absurd situation of a specialty mechanic polishing his

3

small part to a high degree of efficiency without caring whether the whole functions. Specialization is necessary for the purpose of discovery and understanding, and we must continue to study every aspect of being for a better grasp of the whole.

MAN IS MORE THAN A MACHINE

But there is another "must." We must recognize that the whole is greater than the sum of the parts. Man is more than a machine. The understanding and treatment of man's body is body mechanics. Healing is far more. Ours is an age of return to ancient principles, with modern understanding. Today's understanding reveals that *dis-ease*, whether functional, chemical, electrical, or structural in nature, may have its origin in a spiritual distress or may be a result of imbalance in relationships. We can easily demonstrate that a chemical imbalance, if corrected, may reappear or even manifest itself in disguise as a functional or electrical disorder if distress in family relationships or spiritual well-being has not been corrected.

Why should we consider the triune whole? We have no choice. If the very functioning of one special part can be affected by a lack of balance in another, no one can be an authority on a specific part without knowing something of its relationship to those other selves.

An obvious question that arises is, "If the specialists in these rather esoteric areas of mind, emotion, relationships, and spiritual welfare have not agreed upon working hypotheses, how can I hope to benefit by stretching my field beyond those aspects which already are challenging me?"

One answer is that specialists such as ministers and psychiatrists usually are not studying specifically the interface between imbalances in their area of interest and the resulting symptoms in the physical body. There is a great vacuum at the point of interface among the disciplines. But dealing with that interface need not involve esoterics. With more thorough study of these relationships, what seems to be esoteric may become exoteric.

Another question may be, "Isn't this the field of psychosomatic medicine?" Indeed it is, and, in studying it, we are likely to find that there is no dis-ease other than that with psycho-origin. The relatedness of man's components is pervasive.

TEACHER-HEALER-PRIEST

Certainly no wise person would suggest that every physician must become a duly qualified priest or even complete a residency in psychiatry in order to treat his patient adequately. Nor can we reasonably suggest that every pastor must seek a medical degree. Yet it is inescapably true that a pastor is guilty of almost pathologic ignorance should he fail to consider a physiological cause for a parishioner's anxieties. Should not the physician be just as responsible for considering spiritual needs as a possible source of imbalance? The role of teacher is as inescapable for the physician as the role of priest. If he can demonstrate to a patient the relationship between life style and disease or between stressful relationships and disease, then his role as teacher is most effective in any healing he may accomplish.

Thus it appears that the whole physician must accept the challenge of being teacher-healer-priest. He must at least recognize possible sources of disease in ignorance and in spiritual poverty, and must cooperate with family counselors, pastors, nutritionists, and therapists dealing with self-acceptance, consciousness "evolution," music, art, and relaxation.

The whole man is more than the sum of his parts. The sum of the parts is a body with a mind and a spirit. The whole man is a life which includes relationships and communication, as well as the interaction of accomplishments with failures. To treat even the sum of the parts is not really to treat the whole man. Holistic medicine might better be dubbed "synergistic healing," to suggest that adequate treatment may require reaching beyond the body, beyond the mind as we understand it, even beyond the spiritual or religious "body" to explore a patient's relationships, communication, and experiences. Holistic, totalistic, or synergistic healing is far more than body mechanics.

PSYCHOSOMATIC MEDICINE

The concept of psychosomatic medicine is not new. It was described about 3,000 years ago by Moses in the Book of Exodus, and by Solomon in the Book of Proverbs. Both of them understood that a condition of the mind affects the body. Solomon said,

"A cheerful heart is a good medicine, but a downcast spirit dries up the bones" (Proverbs 17:22), meaning perhaps that sadness and bitterness can cause arthritis. That is a statement of psychosomatic medicine.

Before him, Moses had said, "If you will diligently hearken to the voice of the Lord your God, and do that which is right in His sight, and give heed to His commandments and keep all His statutes, I will put none of the diseases upon you which I put upon the Egyptians; for I am the Lord, your healer" (Exodus 15:26). Thus, as the Israelites were coming out of Egypt, they received a promise that, if they were in harmony with their environment, they would not suffer disease. This, too, is a clear statement of psychosomatic medicine. Of course, "psychosomatic" in this sense does not imply that no physical causes or conditions exist. Moses went on to tell his followers that they must eat the right food, wash and purify and boil it, and obey the laws of sanitation, epidemic control, and nutrition. That still comes back to the concept that one's mental outlook and relationships with others and with the environment make one vulnerable to germs and bacteria.

REDEFINING *SPIRITUAL*

As we begin to work together holistically, as we heal the whole, we will understand that prayer and meditation can be effective tools affecting the whole of a person's life, not just spiritual attitudes and relationships. Perhaps we shall redefine the term *spiritual.* Instead of feeling that spiritual growth shows that a person is very religious, perhaps we shall recognize that spiritual growth reflects a person's effectiveness in living. This sort of definition implies that, if a person is not successful at living, neither is he truly spiritual. Spiritual means living in harmony with universal, Divine laws. Then spirituality can very intimately be related to one's bank account, to interpersonal communications, and to physical health, because it reveals the relationship to the whole.

One of the most frightening ideas a helping professional may face is how to deal with a patient's spiritual life. But such a helper *can* do something about a patient's spiritual nature. I want to discuss three aspects in treating the individual. One concerns diagnosis, and one involves the spiritual outlook. Closely related is a third, the X-factor in healing, which I will analyze in the next

THE TRIUNE CONCEPT 7

chapter. All three factors are involved in any real healing situation, whether it involves a physician, a teacher, or a ministerial counselor. The objective in every case is not simply to end symptoms which an individual may have, but to build a new life. This is holism; this is synergism.

When a physician seeks to understand a patient's illness, he usually makes a series of tests. Unfortunately, diagnosis may stop right there. Beyond the tests, apart from the biological functioning, apart from the laboratory findings, is another step in diagnosis. If the physician takes time to understand why the patient is producing certain symptoms in his system and can uncover related factors in his life, we have what is called a *greater diagnosis*. This greater diagnosis often is left out, but, unless the physician makes it, he is treating only one aspect of the patient. The greater diagnosis really occurs when the physician understands the patient, his feelings, and his life through communicating on another level.

THE TWO-SIDED BRAIN

Two kinds of thinking are available to us all the time, but we have been emphasizing one for centuries, and neglecting the other. There are two sides of the brain, and we have developed an intellectual conceit about the method of thinking that we call rational, deductive. We feel we must start with a fact, add to that an observation, then draw a conclusion and gain some information. This, actually, is the more cumbersome approach. There is a second, intuitive side to the brain, and the intuitive process has been discredited. We should find a balance between the two processes, and learn to use both sides of our consciousness. Unless we are using our entire brain, we are not thinking holistically. This means the physician usually must begin with himself by training not only his rational, logical, deductive process in determining what is wrong with a patient, but by learning to ask questions through the intuitive process. This draws from two sources. One is his own higher consciousness, and the other is the patient himself, often the patient's higher consciousness.

Learning to draw upon intuition is part of the meditative process. It is important to clear the mind, to make the rational, deductive mind become quiet, and get in touch with the source of your being. Anyone can begin a dialogue with this source of information by learning to shut up and listen. Simply recognize that there is a greater consciousness than yours and direct your consciousness towards that, towards the source of your being; then ask questions. You will get answers, and this will introduce you to another reality, the other side of consciousness, the right side of your brain, an infinite, inner world which can provide real, usable, practical answers in your life and work.

THE INTUITIVE SENSE

Probably you have not yet learned to use the intuitive sense as skillfully as you use your five physical senses, and you may attribute the answers you begin to get intuitively to your imagination. It is healthy to question any of your senses. How dependable are your eyes? How dependable are your ears? You normally use one sense to verify what another sense is telling you. If you touch something sticky, you quickly open your eyes to check your sense of touch. No sense is completely valid by itself. This is true also of your inner awareness, your intuitive sense. You often have feelings about a person with whom you're working, but, because of your rational, scientific approach, you may dismiss those feelings as "just imagination." Yet, on occasion, you have used this feeling, this intuition. By training this sense, you can make it as valid a tool as any other. This intuitive sense must be checked and validated because information coming from it may be derived from many sources. It can come from ego, from your background and prejudices, or from your education and beliefs. What you receive may not be accurate as it comes until you have learned to understand your intuition and to check it with the other senses.

The process of developing this valuable extra sense, this subtler sense, will take some time, and will require concentration and effort. It is a meditative process, which you can begin by setting aside about twenty minutes each day when you can become quiet, close yourself off from everything else, and practice building for yourself a separate reality. Experience another place of your own choosing. Create for yourself a meadow, a meadow in a valley surrounded by mountains. Feel the grass under your hands, experience the warmth of the sunlight, hear the water in the little brook, and plunge your hand into its cold, swift-moving bubbles. This is visualization, and it becomes consciousness projection when you reach the point where you really *can* put your consciousness in that meadow and be there. Anyone over the age of fourteen may have some difficulty visualizing an experience and making it real because society discourages the use of imagination. However, you can rebuild that tool by practicing visualization to create a meadow which you totally experience. Work on this at home for two or three weeks.

When you really have mastered this consciousness projection, you can begin to do the same thing with those who come to you for healing. You can begin to see and experience and feel what is going on in their bodies. Care enough about a person to take some extra time, to empty your mind of everything else, every other consideration. The person need not be in the room with you. Just focus on that person's image for awhile, and ask within yourself, "What would you like me to know about you? What can you tell me about yourself?" Let images, words, come that can direct you to other levels. You will begin to think of things that never were said verbally.

People often reveal more nonverbally than verbally. Often they are unable to communicate verbally what they wish to say, or are not quite sure that you want to hear it. By learning to listen with another, subtler set of senses, you can gain additional information. The person gives you many signals through body language, and always, in one way or another, he will tell you what is wrong. At some level of consciousness, every person knows exactly what is wrong and the ramifications of his situation—his job, his family, his diet, and everything that affects his condition. He understands why he built it, why he is experiencing it, and why he needs that particular experience. You must learn to listen with the intuitive side of the mind, not to a person's words, but to the source of the words.

When you are able to project your consciousness into the body of a person, you will be drawn instantly to anything wrong. Anything that is not as it should be will attract your attention. You may not see a specific organ or gland, but you may begin to see symbols. If you see red, it probably indicates heat. If you see black or gray or blue, you can assume that the bodily function in that area is depressed or lacking something. Record your feelings and what you think the interpretation might be. Then go ahead with objective tests and see how well they match your intuitive answers. Keep doing this until you have some idea of how valid your intuition may be. As you develop this skill, this ability to learn from your intuition, you will build a bond of caring between yourself and the other person which is an essential part of healing.

IT'S ALL RIGHT TO BE HAPPY!

As you relate to people holistically, on all levels of being, you will recognize another spiritual quality which will help give new life to the person who needs healing. This is not a matter of theology or belief systems or religion. What you can give your patients in the realm of spirit is permission to experience joy. Too often our society frowns upon joy. We actually expect people passing us on the sidewalk to look worried, sad, or dejected, believing that such an expression is normal. If someone dances down the street with a smile spread across his face, everyone turns around to look and wonders, "What's wrong with him?"

Spiritual healing often comes from letting your patient know that it is all right to be deliriously, deliciously happy. There is no reason for not being joyous. The excuses we use for being unhappy are invalid. Being unhappy does not improve a bad situation; it is not an appropriate response. Help people discover whatever they are using to make themselves unhappy. Explore their excuses for not feeling good about themselves. Forget their disease for a moment, forget their specific complaints, and ask, "What things are concerning you most right now? What is worrying you? Are you worried about payments you owe? About your relationships with your family?" If you can learn what these concerns are, either verbally or through your own meditation, try to show the person that being unhappy does not improve the situation. Suggest to him, "Try experiencing joy just because you want to. Decide that you don't need an excuse to be happy, that you aren't dependent upon some person or outside circumstances to make you happy."

Most people don't know that it's all right to be happy when their lives seem full of problems. They think, "As long as these factors are going on, I must be worried. How can I be happy when all these terrible things are happening in the world?" But does being unhappy improve the world, or does being joyous improve the world? Being joyous does make a difference. It is hard to be joyous in a group of people without affecting the entire group. And that is healing. If we can learn to love and laugh, experience and express joy in our lives, if those of us who are healers, ministers, teachers, can demonstrate that we're not worrying, that we are enjoying ourselves and finding a fulfilling life, then we have given an example of encouragement.

WORKING ON YOURSELF

You may need to work on yourself. What makes you depressed, unhappy, worried? What factors cause you to believe that you are a victim of circumstances? You can help people understand that they are not victims, help them to realize that they can be a cause of whatever they experience. But you can do this only if you believe it yourself. You have been the cause all along of what you are experiencing. But you start actively being a cause only when you recognize that you are causing your experience. You must realize that when some stimulus occurs which could hurt your feelings or make you depressed, sad, or frightened, it is *only* a stimulus. The response, the emotion that you experience as a result, is based on your own belief and decision. You can decide how to feel about the situation. If you recognize that, you can choose a different response and become a cause instead of a victim of all that happens in your life. You can decide how you will feel in spite of negative stimuli, and choose joy, happiness, radiant health. Then you will have become a cause, not a victim.

This is a spiritual factor which physicians and healers can use, and religion doesn't limit it at all. People of any religious background can find the source of their being, the causal factor in their lives, the cause of their emotions, the roots of their beliefs, and change whatever is not appropriate. Let them know that it's all right for them to love themselves. If they feel unloved, they probably make themselves unlovely. Many people never got so much attention before they had symptoms. Are you going to take away their symptoms without replacing that attention? One of the healthiest things you can do for people is to teach them that the love they need begins with love for self, self appreciation. It is a revolutionary thought for many people that they deserve to be loved. Help people to realize that they are all right, that they are beautiful. When they know that, they will begin to have what they need to be healed.

2

The X-Factor in Healing

PAUL SOLOMON

We are among the most fortunate people in the world to be witnesses to what God is doing in our generation. This is an especially privileged generation, and we're lucky to be alive now. At a time when many people are saying the world is getting worse and worse, I seem to find a world that's getting better and better and more and more beautiful.

We are approaching the end of medical science as we have known it: the era of chemical drugs and specialization. Medicine now is looking for a new factor in healing that we are only beginning to discover and to put to work. This healing factor goes beyond all the techniques, all the chemical constructs of the physical body, and gives a wholeness to everything. If we discover this healing factor for the individual, it will bring healing to the planet.

Healers of all kinds are practicing many different techniques at the present time. Some are putting their hands on feet, some are putting their hands on heads, some are using music, some are using art, some are using chemicals, and some are using herbs. Some are treating the mind, some are treating the body, and some are treating the spirit. Each, of course, feels that his is the way to do it. How do we synthesize all this? How do we make some practical application?

THE X-FACTOR

I can't tell you what technique to put to work, but I am convinced that, when all of them have been tried, when you have treated the feet and the head, the body and the psyche, corrected the chemical

13

balance and adjusted the vertebrae, you still may not know what factor finally produces healing. Every practitioner knows that when all the adjustments have been made, when the mind has undergone therapy, when the body seems all right, the patient still may not respond. There is an X-factor, something which the techniques, at least, do not reveal. What makes healing work?

Regardless of your practice, your specialty, or your technique, there is a common factor in healing, the single most important factor. It is, in fact, the *one* that makes healing work. You can apply this X-factor through the feet or the head; you can apply it to the body or the mind or the spirit—wherever you find an opening for the person to receive it. But it is this X-factor that will do the healing regardless of the application, regardless of the technique. If this X-factor is not present, you won't heal no matter how well you have mastered your techniques. But, if you do have the X-factor, you probably will heal in spite of your techniques.

I want to describe my discovery of the X-factor. A number of years ago, I had the most spectacular experience of my life, an experience that is just as available to you as it was to me. I discovered that I could communicate with an intelligence that knew far more than I knew, an intelligence that could answer questions, an intelligence that astonished me with the applicability and wisdom of its answers.

Five of us were seeking instructions for healing, and we asked whether we could learn to be healers. Is healing a natural gift that some have and some don't have, or are there techniques which anyone can master to become a healer?

We were told that if we wanted to be healers, each of us should buy two young tomato plants. We should take exactly the same care of the plants, giving each one the same amount of sunlight, water, and food, but we should love one and hate the other. The one we loved would grow and thrive and bear fruit, and the one we hated would wither and die. But when that plant began to wither, we should change our attitude and love it. If we could cause that tomato plant to survive, we could heal human beings with the same energy.

The five of us bought ten tomato plants and set them on my back porch. We gave them sun and water and food. We loved one and hated the other. They all died. We discussed what we might have done wrong, and went back and bought ten more plants, plus a book on the care and feeding of tomatoes. We mixed our soils and tried to be sure that we didn't overwater the plants. Then we loved one and hated the other. They all died.

Three people dropped out of the experiment, but two of us bought two more tomato plants and tried again to do everything right. At this point I was thinking that my dad raises hundreds of tomatoes every summer and sells them by the bushel to make some vacation money. He doesn't love them or hate them or read books about them. He simply puts them out and they grow. It never seemed complicated to raise tomatoes. Why did mine die? So we decided this time not to love one and hate the other, but just to love both. They died anyhow. Two dozen tomato plants were killed! We decided just to ignore the subject of healing for awhile.

But people were coming constantly asking about healing and wanting to know how to participate in healing, and we could not ignore them. One day, I went to a nursery with a friend who wanted to pick up a few plants for his apartment. He and his wife had plants everywhere, like a jungle, and their place was beautiful. I didn't have a single plant in my house. While my friend was selecting a few plants, I was thinking that I would enjoy having some living, growing thing in my house, but I'd probably kill it. Then I saw some tiny cacti growing in little pots, and started to buy two of them. I thought, if they both die, I may never recover; I'll buy two dozen, and they won't all die. So I bought two dozen and created a miniature cactus garden. I thought, I'm not going to love, not going to hate, I'm just going to let them sit there and at least I'll have some plants in my house. I followed instructions about watering them, but as I stopped to check on them from time to time, I made a discovery. I found that I really cared about some of them, that I hoped certain ones would make it, while others didn't matter especially.

Suddenly I realized that I never really had loved or hated any of the tomato plants. I had been doing an experiment, and my attention was on myself, not the tomatoes. I cared whether I succeeded, not whether the plants survived. That is not love, and that does not heal. Genuine caring is the quality that makes the difference. That was my greatest lesson: a conjured love will not heal. Real love, a heartfelt love, makes the difference, and enables healing to occur. The X-factor in healing is love.

THE COMMUNITY IN THE DESERT

About two thousand years ago, in the Jordanian desert, there lived some people who discovered this same law. It was a period when those who seemed to have a communicable disease were just put outside the city gates so they wouldn't infect anyone and were left there to die. Anyone who cared about them left scraps of food outside the gates, so that the sick might come to get it and carry it off to wherever they were trying to survive.

But in this special community hidden in the desert, were a few people who cared more than that. Their teachers had told them, "If you want to heal, what you really are asking is to give life to another person. The only way to give life to another is to give your own life to another, and be prepared to care for him for the rest of his days if necessary."

A spectacular thing happened. When they brought the sick people from the city gates, and cared for them awhile, they found that, when they gave their lives to this care, the sick often recovered in short order. These healers learned not only to give themselves. They discovered the therapeutic value of hot sand from the desert for increasing circulation; they discovered the therapeutic value of cold spring water; they discovered the value of herbs and spices, and they became herbalists. They traveled a great deal, and became known in many lands as Therapeutae, the Greek word for "healers." But, in many places, they found that what they needed for healing was not at hand. They couldn't carry hot sand in a bag and keep it hot, nor cold spring water and keep it cold. The important thing they learned was that, when they stopped to treat the sick, if what they most needed was not at hand, they could substitute something else. If they needed hot sand, and there was none, they could pick leaves off a tree and tell them to do what hot sand would do. They had learned to apply the laws of healing, and, by obeying the law, they had overcome the law and the law obeyed them. What really made the difference in their healing was that they loved enough to give a life to healing. Techniques are useful, but they are nothing more than a system of exchange for moving energy. None of the techniques matters except as a method for transferring that which does matter, which is love in the heart of the healer.

The Scripture says that God is love. God heals. Love heals. If you love someone, you "God" someone. Love is the original force, the first cause, the energy from which all matter is created. This is life force, the breath of God. The Gospel of John begins by saying, "In the beginning was the word, and the word was with God, and the word was God." The Greek for *word* is "logos," and *logos* can be translated as "expression" instead of *word*. We can say, "In the beginning, God expressed Himself." That expression was love, and He made the world out of it. This is the one prime force, the energy flowing through all matter. As it moved in the beginning, it resulted in form. If we move it again, we can change the form that resulted from it.

HEALING AND LOVING

That is what healing is about. There are two steps to healing. One is to love in order to move energy, and the other is to move love into a particular shape or form, changing a condition so that it manifests itself in another way. Before you can do any effective healing, you must do some effective loving.

In the first chapter, we saw that a physician can learn to make a greater diagnosis based upon intuition, upon caring enough to be alone in consciousness with a patient for a few moments in order to build the bond that will allow healing to occur. The period of meditation, of trying to receive thoughts from the patient, should be done even if you don't need to have such information for diagnosis. Its purpose is to form that bond through which you can communicate, through which you can give him the energy that would heal your own body if you needed healing. This energy, this vitality, will supplement the patient's ability to overwhelm the disease within him. If you can listen and get valid information about what is going on in his body, then you have an indication that you have formed a bond, made contact with the consciousness of that patient. Then watch how your relationship changes.

You have a healing, growing life-energy moving through you that is available for healing in your own body. It can be lent from you to another. I am convinced that if it cannot heal your body, then something is wrong with your *self* love. The X-factor in healing is love, and that is not just love for another; it is love for oneself as well. Any doctor knows that, if a patient is happy, he'll heal faster. If he likes his job, he'll heal faster. If he's getting along with his family, he'll heal faster. If he cares for himself and his life, loves who he is and what he is, that love will heal him. And love can move from one person to another.

Many healers draw attention to themselves and say, "Look at me! I'm a healer!" At almost any conference you attend, you see someone with his hand on another person and the other hand in the air. Who is drawing energy? How is attention being conveyed to the patient? To heal, you must care more about what the patient is thinking than what you are thinking, must give up for a moment your opinions, thoughts, ideas, and begin to experience those of the patient. Your attention, love, and concern must be on him instead of yourself. Then the healing life force that is in you can go to him. Where your consciousness is, your energy will follow.

THE LAYING-ON-OF-HANDS

A beautiful lady in New York named Delores Krieger did extensive research on laying-on-of-hands healing. She was a professor of nursing at New York University. In her experiments, she worked with control groups of nurses to see if she could prove whether laying-on-of-hands made a difference in healing. She did discover that laying-on-of-hands can affect the hemoglobin count in the blood, but that did not always promote healing. She wanted to find the variables: when did healing occur and when didn't it?

She tested nurses who were religious, but they could do no better. She tested nurses with more vitality, but that made no difference. She ran out of criteria until one day a nurse told her, "You know, I hope this works for Miss So-and-So; I really *care* about her!" Then she tested that additional factor: caring. She discovered that the variable which made the most difference was whether a nurse *cared* for a particular patient. Again, the X-factor in healing was love.

LOVE THEM BECAUSE THEY *ARE*

If you want to become a healer, don't move from chemistry to herbs, from one kind of therapy to another. Move to caring specifically and individually about a person. The greatest need of most people who come to you is to know that somebody in this world loves them. Not many people are absolutely certain that they are loved. They feel insecure about being loved. If you can show them that you love them, not because they have symptoms, but because they *are*, then you can help them to love themselves. Our culture teaches us as we grow up that it's not all right to love ourselves. But there is a creative power that went to great trouble to put together the very delicate instruments we inhabit. What right has any of us to reject our body by saying, "This old thing isn't much!" We should appreciate the beauty, the intricacy, the delicacy of the instruments that have been given us. If we know that we are beautiful, it is easier for us to notice that others are beautiful. If we are confident that we are all right, then we don't need to compete with one another, and it is easier to notice that others are all right as well, because they don't threaten us.

As a healer, you must love your patients without being afraid that they will reject you. Become secure enough to feel for each person a love that does not depend on whether the person follows your advice. It does not depend on whether he performs satisfactorily or whether he returns your love. If you can love that freely, you can heal. With that sort of nourishment and support, the body and the psyche can overcome almost any other enemy. If you can give love in large doses, you will find healing happening.

This is loving impersonally, loving each individual, not because of anything he can return to you personally, but because he is an expression of God. Too often love is a selfish force that tries to manipulate others. We say we love someone, but we mean we are investing our happiness in that person, and we will be hurt if our love is not returned. Impersonal love goes a step beyond; it is not conditional upon any obligation or return. This sort of love is the prime creative force in the universe; this is the love that heals. When we begin to discover that all things in the universe cooperate with the force that created them and are subject to that energy, we can live in harmony with all life and with all power. Finding the source of life within your own being, learning to invoke and to cooperate with that, allows you to use it to help all other things, to live in harmony with your environment. It will allow you to produce harmony in the lives of others, to heal.

HARMONY WITH THE FORCES OF LIFE

It would be a good idea, when entering your place of work each morning, to touch everything that you will use and invoke its co-operation in producing the results you seek. That kind of thought, that kind of invocation and harmony with the forces of life around you, will produce harmony within you. Once you have become master of your own being and the forces within you, you will find other forces around you beginning to respond—your healing abilities, your associates, your tools, and the life forces of those whom you contact for healing.

This is the energy which will change the nature of mankind. It may be discovered in the field of health; it may be discovered in the field of education, or of religion. Wherever it is discovered and put to work at its full capacity, it will bring about a transmutation from the old heaven and earth to a new heaven and earth. It will bring healing not only to individuals, but to the planet.

3

*Why People Must Manage Their Own Health Care**

LAWRENCE L. WEED

The "scientific approach" to solving problems is a set of rules to reduce mistakes and increase benefits as we interpret our observations and the results of our actions. The rules are commonplace and easy to understand. They are not always easy to follow in complex situations such as the interactions between patients and health care providers. Review of some of the rules quickly reveals why the patients themselves must become actively involved; it is the only way we shall control the overuse and misuse of drugs and procedures and the rising costs in the medical care system.

Variables:

The more variables you know and consider in a situation, the wiser you can be in that situation. The more continuous the observation of the variables, the smoother the necessary adjustments can be.

In maintaining health, in chronic disease, and in the events that lead to acute illness, the patients themselves know and control more of the relevant variables than anyone else. Patients live with the variables all the time. When the values of those variables change (when the situation changes), they can be the first to know.

Physicians often know only a few of the variables and usually

* Adapted with permission from "Your Health Care and How To Manage It", by Lawrence L. Weed, M.D. (1975). Distributed by PROMIS Laboratory, University of Vermont, Burlington, Vermont, 05401.

21

have direct control over none. Physicians and other medical personnel see a fragment of the total during a fragment of the time.

Examples:

1. *Managing Variables in a Chronic Disease.* In a diabetic in which we use the blood sugar level as a goal and index of control, the following variables are some that are known to affect it:

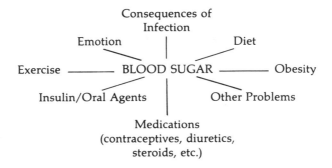

2. Understanding and managing variables that predispose to acute disease:

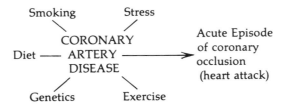

The patient is aware of and has control over more of the above variables than anyone else. The physician goes to medical school and tries to learn textbook averages about many diseases. The patient knows many things that the disease does to him; the facts are his with no formal education at all.

Therefore:

Responsibility for health care rests in the patient's hands because that is where the knowledge of and control of the variables lie. To meet this responsibility, the patient needs:

1. The conviction that it is his responsibility to look at the variables and to act upon them. Previous data on similar patients can give some guidance, but only his own exact past data can tell him what adjustments must be made. This has to be so because no two people are exactly the same combination of variables.
2. The correct tools and guidance to interpret and act upon the variables wisely.
3. Above all the patient needs the responsibility itself; otherwise a dependency state is created, self-respect is lost, motivation diminishes, and the patient withdraws—leaving the situation to professional providers who cannot control or even know about many of the variables.

Variables and Records:

Keeping track of variables over time and examining for crucial inter-relationships are beyond the capacity of the unaided human mind. Records are necessary.

Patients can capitalize upon their awareness of and continuous exposure to most of the variables by learning to keep and read their own records, including graphs and flowsheets. They can discern their own unique patterns of response and be the first to see what works and what does not work. The data can protect them from their own unfounded notions and from the misconceptions and generalizations of those who treat them.

Furthermore, they will not charge for keeping the record, they will not run out of storage room, there will be one medical librarian for each record in the country, and accessibility/retrieval problems as the patient moves around should be minimal. Patients will not have to repeat their story and explain what pills and tests they have had every time they see a new medical person. They will not always have to be wondering whether the physician or nurse knows all he should as he starts new and serious treatments. Patients and society will not have to pay the bill for all the inefficiencies that result from the redundancies and poor communication in the medical profession.

Providers specialize and a single patient is treated by more than one specialist. Each specialist keeps a separate record for each patient, and each patient is unaware of that record's contents; therefore, crucial information is not readily available when it is needed. When institutions run out of storage space and money for proper record maintenance, the patient pays for the confusion and lack of availability of needed information.

When patients visit the office of a specialist or when they are admitted to a hospital, including the academic medical centers, it is not the custom to simply add the necessary new information and plans to a single, cumulative account of the individual's health status. Much of the information from physicians' offices and personal memories is not even available, let alone organized in a form common to all. Rather, patients are "worked-up" from scratch repeatedly, and this process takes hours of extra time; providers often skip crucial information from past records as a result. There is no good system whereby efforts are cumulative and coordinated; the result is that the right hand does not know what the left hand is doing. Some physicians try to solve the problem by extreme dedication and overwork, but they frequently end up disillusioned and dissatisfied. This is particularly true of house officers who may admit as many as five patients in one evening, each with a few words scribbled on a prescription blank from the person who sent them in. Since providers do not simply add to a single, complete, organized, cumulative record, the house officer stays up all night and, even then, does not get the job done properly. Furthermore, there is a tradition in doctor training and practice to do your "night on" alone no matter what the load. Support from second and third back-up call systems is not used so that patients can be guaranteed adequate attention. The patient admitted alone on one night with a thoughtful superior doctor is in very different circumstances from the one admitted with five other patients on the same night when all are under the care of a less skilled physician. Patients and families of patients must be aware of these realities so that they can begin to mobilize cumulative accounts of their own situation and actively help the providers bring the information under control.

Also, because coordination is so bad, logic so poorly preserved in the written record, and medical personnel rely so much on fallible human memories for information on patients and medical knowledge, intelligent analysis of medical action on populations of patients is all but impossible on a routine basis. Many of our mistakes go undetected. Occasionally, a disease like Legionnaires' disease will erupt and the government will spend thousands of dollars trying to piece together past actions from scattered, disorganized, and illegible records which were never checked for quality in the first place. Or occasionally an academic person will study a subject like antibiotic use and find, as they recently published in an article from Duke University, that 64% of the time the wrong antibiotic is given or the wrong dose is used. How much worse does medicine have to get before the medical establishment realizes and admits that there is something wrong with this disorganized, memory-based, uncoordinated, inefficient system for communication and problem solving?

Therefore:

The patient must have a copy of his own record. He must be involved with organizing and recording the variables so that the course of his own data on disease and treatment will slowly reveal to him what the best care for him should be. Crippling dependency states in patients will be fewer. Needless repetition of expensive and dangerous medical activities will be controlled.

It is true that there are those who live to a ripe, old age, are rarely sick, have handled what medical problems they have with natural body defenses and no medical records. Compulsive thinking about health and medical record keeping could do more harm to them than good. We can certainly let them continue in the successful medical approaches they have worked out for themselves. But for those who are not always healthy and have not found personal approaches that work for them and who continuously turn to the medical profession for guidance, and upon whom actions are taken and records kept (good and bad), we are merely saying that these individuals must get involved, must understand the actions and records, and must study the results of the interventions. Otherwise, they could be victims of some of the bad effects that disorganized medical activity can generate.

Relationships Among Variables:

Scientists record and observe the course of variables to look for trends and associations among them. To separate coincidence from cause and effect, they observe many times and use mathematical techniques to analyze. Some relationships are simple to see; every time the temperature gets low the water freezes; others are more subtle. Scientists hypothesize and manipulate variables to bring out relationships, but they try to change one at a time so they will know what is causing what. They do not draw conclusions beyond what the data will support.

In medicine, particularly in chronic disease, the patient continually lives with the variables and knows better than anyone else when many, not just one, are changing. He knows that conclusions about what is causing what should be made with great caution. At the present time patients have little access to the data and the physician's thought processes. In their ignorance of these facts and with unfounded expectations for an "instant cure," they develop exaggerated ideas of the physician's power and demand diagnostic conclusions at times when none are possible. In an honest medical setting, none are possible much more than half the time. Patients need to be taught a tolerance of ambiguity; it can be tolerated when they have access to the data and the physician's logic concerning their problems.

Physicians and other medical providers are away from the patients and the variables most of the time. They write an order to change one variable like an insulin dose and assume the others to be constant (which they rarely are). It is very common for the very same physicians who fail to get enough data or to organize the variables at the outset to also be the ones who introduce too many new, uncontrolled variables (excessive ordering of laboratory tests, procedures, and drugs). Furthermore they analyze and interpret the results either inadequately or sometimes not at all; they needlessly change too many variables at once, and draw conclusions from uncontrolled situations and from numbers of cases that are not statistically significant. The pressure from uninformed patients for diagnosis and predictions increases these tendencies among providers.

Even when physicians change just one variable in the analysis of one problem, they may completely ignore the effects of that change on the other problems. Furthermore, many physicians try to deal with all this complexity in their heads—without good records, without carefully constructed flowsheets and graphs; there is no organization of data to help them avoid mistakes, and without such organized data, they may fail to recognize their own mistakes. Their confidence goes on undisturbed.

Therefore:

Patients must know what providers are thinking, what they are trying to do or demonstrate, what the variables are so that they can protect the provider and themselves from invalid conclusions. Good science and good medicine are not just accurate data, not just a lot of data, and not just a brilliant analysis of some of the data. They are all three, and it takes a cooperative approach with adequate tools to achieve all three. Records cannot do it alone, providers cannot do it alone, patients cannot do it alone, and guidance tools cannot do it all alone. They must be coupled into a smoothly working unit. It is not "The Record," "My Doctor," "That Computer"—it is the right combination to identify and solve the problem.

The right combination is very difficult to achieve consistently. That is why massive expenditures on specialized parts of the body do not achieve massive improvements in mortality and morbidity statistics. Matters could get worse because even the marvelous balancing mechanisms of nature that have evolved over millions of years cannot keep up with the uncontrolled interventions of increasing numbers of people who make their living manipulating variables in the general population, all in the name of "medical care."

The medical schools are the worst offenders. They teach and examine for facts out of all proportion to teaching and examining for the capacity to collect and organize data effectively, control variables, and draw conclusions rigorously. The transmission of the medical school faculty's scientific facts often overwhelms—even precludes—the transmission of scientific behavior to students. The failures in medical education are, in their own way, every bit as bad as the failures in grade school education that are now so widely discussed. Discipline and follow through on medical actions are largely absent in much of medical practice today. The simple principles taught in the sixth grade general science courses are violated day after day in patient care. Patients must understand that even if medical schools were to change tomorrow (and they will not), it would be years before that change would help them.

THE SCIENTIFIC PRINCIPLES ARE SIMPLE, AND YOU CAN APPLY THEM TO YOURSELF IMMEDIATELY IN YOUR OWN THINKING ABOUT YOUR OWN MEDICAL CARE. STOP EXPECTING THE "IMPOSSIBLE" FROM THE MEDICAL PROFESSION AND START DOING THE "POSSIBLE" FOR YOURSELF.

Variables From Mind and Body:

Variables in real problems do not follow the boundaries of academic disciplines. Identifying as many relevant variables as possible should precede the analysis and manipulation of the few variables that are easily seen and understood by the specialist.

In health and disease there is no boundary line between the mind and the body. The patients naturally see the flow from one to the other. It is common to hear them say: "She comes home with tummy aches when she has that teacher." "He's continually fighting with his boss; he better watch his blood pressure." "The in-laws hadn't been there two days when she had a migraine and an asthmatic attack."

Physicians divide themselves into psychiatric services, medical services, surgical services, etc. The flow of mind-body relationships is often not perceived across their man-made boundaries. The work-up for the back pain on the orthopedic service looks completely different from the work-up for the back pain on the psychiatric service.

You are in the best position to keep data that could reveal true cause and effect relationships among mental and physical events. Physicians and other providers may be either paternalistic and draw conclusions and make judgments on only a few of the variables and without consultation with you, the patient; or they may act too hastily on undocumented, verbal, anecdotal notions of patients about cause and effect.

Therefore:

Providers must encourage the patient to keep his own data; the provider must share all the data he has and must review his interpretations with the patient so that the patient in turn can critically review what is being done and accept the obligation of changing it if he does not understand or agree. And, if the providers do not encourage or offer to share and review, then patients must demand the information.

A goal should be to let the data speak to both the patient and the provider and have record keeping tools to accomplish that.

We do not need compulsive documentation of the normal, daily interactions, but when troubles and problems appear, we must not improvise hasty solutions from the patient's or doctor's memory.

Motivation Versus Knowledge:

Really wanting to know and taking the time to find out are what lead to scientific advances and a body of knowledge and understanding.

In their own health problems, people are naturally motivated to ask questions and seek answers. They can also solve problems if they are given the proper tools and enough time, even if their knowledge is deficient at the outset. Knowledge help is found all over once you start to look for it—in public libraries, the latest edition of the Encyclopedia Britannica, pamphlets of all sorts from numerous agencies and many departments of the federal government. The individual's own medical record is the basic tool he needs to organize and pursue the problems and the information related to them.

PHYSICIANS AND OTHER PROVIDERS ARE NOT NATURALLY MOTIVATED TO ASK QUESTIONS AND STATE PROBLEMS FROM THE PATIENT'S POINT OF VIEW. THEY CONTINUALLY SEE THINGS IN TERMS OF THE WAY THEY WERE TRAINED AND THE SPECIALTY THEY ENTERED. This gives them the skill and drive necessary to solve a problem in their area once it is presented, but it does not lead them to naturally organize and review all the problems and set priorities from the patient's point of view.

Therefore:

Patients must be educated in the use of tools such as the problem-oriented record and computerized Problem Oriented Medical Record so that there is some concrete instrument for expressing and capitalizing upon their own motivation. If the patients are not motivated enough to use the tools effectively, then we should get over the illusion that those same patients are accomplishing much with twenty minute visits to providers or that they are complying very precisely with directions from those providers, except in those instances where a normally healthy individual gets specialized care for a self-limited problem from the appropriate specialist, e.g. a broken leg.

The Power of the Right Tools:

Tools extend our muscles, our senses, our memories, and our analytical capacities. Extending our muscles and our senses with automobiles, power tools, telescopes, etc. are commonplace. Extending our basically chemical and electronic minds with electronic computers is becoming more commonplace.

For patients who, up until now, have had little exposure in school or elsewhere to the use of the medical record as a powerful tool in their own health care, the particular form of this tool will be of little consequence so long as it is clear to them and usable by them. A computerized problem-oriented record will not be any newer or more confusing to them than traditional paper records since they never had either record in the past.

Physicians, nurses, and other providers have been trained with a whole set of habits and notions about medical records and their availability to patients. It is difficult for some of them to switch to electronic tools that provide specific guidance for solving problems within the context of patients' other problems. Some not only do not want to switch to an electronic record system, they still do not recognize that the record should be a tool for the patient's use as much as a tool for their own use.

Therefore:

In health care, patients and very inexpensive paramedical people who are already a permanent part of a community must be taught to use the problem solving guidance in their own records and eventually in computers. After all, rescue squads with remarkable skill in heart and lung disease have been developed all over the country, and people with only a high school education or less have been taught to do sophisticated medical work. Surely we all can learn to deal with many of the less life-threatening disorders such as sore throats and body aches if we have our records and the right guidance tools. Expensively trained medical professionals should be reserved for specialized tasks that we cannot master and cannot do for ourselves. They also should be used to build the guidance in the tools and to monitor occasionally our records and behaviors to make sure that we are behaving in a disciplined and reliable manner.

Uniqueness:

Multiple variables, constantly changing, continuously create unique combinations. If one hundred different people were each to drive from New York to Los Angeles, we could not predict accurately their exact routes. A road map of the United States shows all the major towns and an enormous number of highways connecting them. The map facilitates travel—the unique requirements of the traveler determine which of the many paths is chosen.

Every patient is a unique traveler through the medical landscape. There are no two patients—even with the same disease—who have the same manifestations, the same course, and the same qualitative and quantitative constellation of accompanying problems. Nor do they have the same goals and same resources to reach those goals. But, just as the same map can be given to and used by many travelers, so the best medical options can be given to each person as he and the provider slowly work their way, step by step, through a medical or social problem.

Determining the best regimen for an individual in chronic disease and the best program for prevention for what appears to be just acute, episodic disease (e.g., the perforated ulcer) is always a matter of research because of the uniqueness of individuals.

Patterns of Uniqueness: Although a patient is unique, his unique patterns of illness and response to treatment tend to repeat themselves in recurrences of a given disease and even in different diseases. In other words, how a patient gets sick is more related to his constitutional background and habits than to the outside agent causing his illness. Expose a group of people to the same amount of virus or bacterial agent or a simple ankle injury and notice the extremely broad spectrum of responses. The patient has only his problem or problems to be concerned with and years to master his responsibilities.

Physicians and other medical providers and scientists have organized medical knowledge in terms of diseases, emphasizing those manifestations of the disease that are common to the largest number of people with the disease. In medical care review they divide people up into groups of people with a given disease and look for common findings and treatments in judging the care of a disease. When medical plans and procedures are ordered, they are frequently done on the basis of this medical knowledge in medical textbooks. Frequently, the medical knowledge about the unique patient kept in the individual patient record is ignored in favor of textbook averages. Medical care is too often not tailored to an individual's unique needs as defined by his previously recorded, unique patterns.

Therefore:

The patient must understand his uniqueness if he is to understand why he must have a primary role in his own care and if he is to control his unrealistic expectations. The patient must understand that, because he is unique, the results of any medical intervention cannot be predicted with absolute confidence. Follow-through and adjustments are everything as the data unfold. The patient, it is true, may not do his part, but at least we can get him over the illusion that anyone can do it for him. For many aspects of management, a physician's partially-recalled knowledge cannot possibly compete with a patient's organized knowledge of himself. Our job is to give the patient the tools and responsibility to organize the knowledge and slowly learn to integrate it. This can be done with modern guidance tools.

The patient must be made aware of the above principle and its implications for his responsibility in his own care. He must first think through the past and then tell those helping him what he thinks the future course will be on the basis of his detailed knowledge of his past reactions and behaviors. Uninformed providers now discover things through painful experiences and unnecessary trial and error. They also draw the wrong conclusions from the limited, parochial variables they so painstakingly analyze. Specialization and limiting the patient's role suppress whole series of variables that profoundly affect outcomes.

Time and Achievement:

Most scientists seek a certain level of achievement, and they adjust the time spent and the number of tasks attempted accordingly. To the extent that a non-fiction writer misjudges his own work, the editor of the journal is expected to judge it further, and if it is not up to a certain standard, it is sent back for further work or further drafts. The amount of time the investigator has spent or the number of other things he is working on count for nothing in the evaluation of the work.

Among people both sick and well, there are no two who will take the same time to master their responsibilities in their own health care. Unfortunately, in all of their education, they have been treated as if people are equal and should arrive at the same standards in the same time. They took the same number of courses over the same number of school years. When the results were different, instead of saying "the data show us our system is wrong" (some require more time than others to do things correctly), we said "some are better or worse than others," gave grades and prizes, punishment and disgrace and drove them all on to the next step leaving a trail of tasks done poorly.

Physicians and other providers often make *time* the constant and *achievement* the variable with patients. They try to do everything for the patient themselves and even keep all the records to themselves and instruct the patients hurriedly over a series of timed appointments. They do not have the time or money to give the necessary time to those who need it; on the other hand, they also have patients who return for repeated office visits that are unnecessary because those patients understood their situation at the first visit and can manage their own affairs. In such medical practices the patient is not only being denied his essential role as an informed participant in his care, he is also being denied the basis to form an accurate judgment about the quality of health care he is purchasing.

Therefore:

Responsibility for quality must, in large part, rest with the patient. A patient can make time the variable in his own health care and stick to something until it is mastered, once he is given the responsibility to do so—like working out the right insulin dosage. A provider must audit until the necessary result is achieved and must avoid over-involvement when he is no longer needed.

THE ART OF MEDICINE:
COMPASSION AND SCIENTIFIC PRINCIPLES

Compassion and Responsibility:

The most compassionate thing to do in the long run is to do things right. For all the common sense reasons and scientific reasons given above, each individual has to do much for himself if the right things are ever to be done. The most effective way to be responsible to others is first of all to be responsible for ourselves and not be a burden to others. We can show our compassion for others by helping them be independent. Compassion that creates dependency states in others is a misguided compassion that demoralizes and destroys.

The Art of Medicine:

Finally you may ask where does the *art* of medicine fit in? Surely no system will make one kind, thoughtful, or sympathetic: to care deeply about the plight of others is a quality not dispensed in manuals of any type. But to say that the art of medicine is not dependent on a great deal of discipline and order is to miss perhaps the true understanding of what underlies art in any form. The physician as well as the musician and poet should read the following words of Stravinsky and at least recognize the possibility that they also apply to him:

> A mode of composition that does not assign itself limits becomes pure fantasy. The effect it produces may accidentally amuse, but is not capable of being repeated. The creator's function is to sift the elements he receives, for human activity must impose limits upon itself. The more art is controlled, limited, worked over, the more it is free. . . .

> As for myself, I experience a sort of terror when, at the moment of setting to work and finding myself before the infinitude of possibilities that present themselves, I have the feeling that everything is permissible to me. If everything is permissible to me, the best and the worst; if nothing offers me any resistance, then any effort is inconceivable, and I cannot use anything as a basis, and consequently, every undertaking becomes futile. . . .

> What delivers me from the anguish into which an unrestricted freedom plunges me is the fact that I am always able to turn immediately

to the concrete things that are here in question. I have no use for a theoretic freedom. Let me have something finite, definite—matter that can lend itself to my operation only insofar as it is commensurate with my possibilities. And such matter presents itself to me together with its limitations. I must in turn impose mine upon it. So here we are, whether we like it or not, in the realm of necessity. And yet which of us has ever heard talk of art as other than a realm of freedom? This sort of heresy is uniformly widespread because it is imagined that art is outside the bounds of ordinary activity. Well, in art as in everything else, one can build only upon a resisting foundation: whatever constantly gives way to pressure constantly renders movement impossible. . . .

My freedom thus consists in my moving about within the narrow frame that I have assigned myself for each one of my undertakings.[1]

4

Using Inner and Outer Resources

PETER ALBRIGHT

Self-development toward the goals of individual responsibility and vibrant health is, as much as anything else, an educational process in which people learn to tune in to various signals and to adjust their lives accordingly. In this process, they activate and refine certain skills which enable them to function well in a self-directed health maintenance program.

The signals which point the way come from many different sources. A source of the greatest importance is the individual's own body. Through the many marvelous, natural biofeedback mechanisms which are part of the cosmic design of our bodies, we derive information, much of it instantaneous, which directs our activities. A simple example of this is the heat of a fire which tells the sensors in our finger to move away to a safer location!

Other signals from which we learn come from beyond the five physical senses. Much is written and studied about this under the headings of ESP, extended sensory perception, higher sense perception, radiesthesia, dowsing, and others. Sensitivity to signals in this realm is thought by some to be possessed by only a few special people, but this is not true; nearly everyone has this capacity, and it can be developed through use.

A very important source of information is tapped by reading and listening to the words of those who are in touch with the ancient and rediscovered wisdom. In the past few years, there has been an explosion of books, conferences, and workshops in the area of self-development, and it only remains to pick and choose what one is to learn.

SOME STEPS TO TAKE

Self-healing and the maintenance of health depend on the judicious use of inner and outer resources. Certain steps must be taken and certain elements must be present before these processes become operational. A first step is becoming comfortable and confident about using and relying on one's inner resources. A way of starting on this path is to study how other people have already learned to depend on their inner resources. To do this, one might read about someone's experiences or attend a workshop or a course.

In the particular area of the search for alternatives to orthodox health care, many people have found obstacles in their path. Worth mentioning in this connection are the high value placed in some circles on conformity and a related resistance to accepting alternative ideas and methods. When these attitudes recede to a lower level of intensity, people will feel much more relaxed about pursuing alternative courses. Of the greatest importance here is an attitude of open-mindedness about concepts and ideas (which is always accompanied by an especially low level of anxiety about being exposed to something new). This will inevitably lead to our being open to each other's needs.

Having observed the value derived by other people from depending on their own resources, one can then proceed to develop inner strengths to an optimal level. Through this process, confidence continues to grow. Again, conferences, workshops, and reading in selected areas are useful tools. A kind of community resource just developing as a means of giving people this information is the holistic health center. The center characteristically devotes much energy to assisting people in the development of these skills, which include selecting a diet high in energy and low in toxicity, adopting the optimal program for exercising and resting the body, and finding the best method of achieving a serene consciousness of the inner and higher self.

OUTSIDE HELPERS

Eventually, an important point is reached when we begin to realize that there are limits to the ability to cope with life situations without the help of other people, even though inner abilities may be developed to a very high level. The next step is to learn how a person's inner strengths for healing and maintenance of health can be fortified by all sorts of helpers from the outside world. The same kinds of learning experiences are available here as in the previous steps.

This leads into a vital area, where the enhancement of certain skills and abilities already present can produce a very high level of functioning within the holistic system. Continuing along this path, one will learn to increase judgment and discernment through the exercise of intuition and logical reasoning, thereby increasing the ability to know how and when to seek and use outside resources to assist the inner forces of healing and maintenance of health. The development of such discernment is a key to the ability to assume more responsibility for one's own health in a safe and competent manner.

There are those currently writing in scientific journals[1] about what they see as the problems of self-responsibility with which the holistic approach is attempting to "burden" people. It is clear that people must not be encouraged to take responsibility for which they are not prepared or of which they are not capable. It does seem, however, that, if a general plan is followed similar to what is outlined in this chapter, the limits of one's abilities will gradually become clear, and the amount of outside help needed will soon become apparent.

CHANGES IN EDUCATION

There is a corollary to the ideas and the process we have been discussing. It is clear that people who already have knowledge and experience in the healing arts should be encouraged and enabled to create optimal ways for others to acquire the knowledge they seek for their own healing and health maintenance. This goal can be met in a number of ways. Our society needs effective public education to counteract the effects of the negative programming which is so prevalent. Bets Albright's article in the next section deals with this situation in detail.

Those in orthodox medical practice ought to be urged to augment the amount and quality of their patients' education. The formation of holistic health centers should be encouraged, since this is an optimal atmosphere in which to teach the principles of self-responsibility and decision-making in relation to health. All other forms of education and research in the area of personal responsibility for health maintenance should be supported. The people of today's world have shown an appetite for understanding and looking after themselves with appropriate help from other people.

This is a healthy reaction to what has gone before. In the next section, we will look at the standard health care system in use today, and we will see how the present-day philosophy of health care developed. We will also see why many people are now looking to holistic healthcare to supply their need to feel vibrantly healthy.

PART II
Sickness and Health: The Conventional Wisdom and How We Got It

5

The Scientific Method and the Medical Model

PETER ALBRIGHT

A large majority of the health care in today's Western world is based on the Western medical model, which is based in turn on the scientific method. This chapter will explore the origins and development of healthcare in our society so that we can better understand the past accomplishments and inherent merits, as well as the limitations and deficiencies, of the Western medical philosophy and system. In this way, we can begin to see why holistic health care is developing as an alternative to—perhaps a replacement for—the medical model.

Let us first consider the scientific method, which was developed for measuring, recording, and interpreting certain kinds of information, originally in the physical realm, but more recently in other areas, such as the realm of energy. For example, we have seen Einstein hypothesizing the interrelationship of mass and energy, and then working out the proof, which other scientists in the field were able to confirm with their own experiments. These events played a big part in the development of post-Newtonian physics.

Many people were involved in the development of the scientific method over the centuries. At least as far back as 3000 B.C., the Egyptians and Babylonians were working on studies in anatomy and physiology, mathematics, geometry, measurements, the calendar, and systems of numbers. A little later, the Chinese developed their own systems of writing and mathematics, making advances in astronomy, chemistry, and medicine. For many centuries, the primitive nature of communications did not permit scientists and scholars in the East and the West to influence each other.

Some mystery attaches to the scientific method, because even scientists have difficulty being sure of the sequence of the steps used by the mind in solving problems. Many scientists believe that the mind does not solve problems in a systematic way, but that it can go back and analyze the problem and the solution once the problem has been solved.

Many people now feel that the use of intuition is involved in the way problems are solved. Critics of this theory argue that previously learned and stored information is the source of this intuition, while others believe in a universal pool of information which we all share on a subconscious level and which we can tap into at any time, provided we learn a method for doing so.

ANALYZING THE SCIENTIFIC METHOD

In any event, regardless of how and at what point the scientist acquires an idea or a bit of information or insight, he may use the scientific method to develop the information further. At least five steps in the process are usually described. Let us use an *example* to illustrate the five steps. In this example, the idea that we hand to the scientist is: *to utilize nuclear fission to produce usable energy.*

Step 1. Stating the problem:

There is a worldwide need for a new source of energy to replace the depleted and rapidly vanishing reserves of fossil fuel. The problem then is: how can one develop a new method of producing usable energy for heat, light, communication, transportation, etc.?

Step 2. Forming a hypothesis:

In this case, the statement of the hypothesis might be: By setting up a nuclear reactor which will boil water and operate a steam turbine, electricity might be produced in a practical and satisfactory manner, thereby creating a suitable replacement for the vanishing supplies of fossil fuel.

Step 3. Observing and experimenting:

In this stage, one constructs a model generating-system, and discovers a number of observable facts, including the following:

a. Nuclear energy can indeed be transformed into electrical energy by this method.
b. In actual practice, when all of the costs are considered and added up, the method proves to be quite expensive.
c. It turns out to be very difficult to construct a generating plant which can contain the radioactivity of the process under all operating conditions.
d. There are radioactive by-products of the process from which the population must be protected for 250,000 years.
e. It is observed that the natural sources of uranium, the fuel for the process, are exhaustible, just as are the fossil fuels.

Step 4. Interpreting the data:

It appears from the data gathered that, while electricity can be generated by this method, it results in neither a safe, economical, nor permanent solution of the problem.

Step 5. Drawing conclusions:

It appears that a better solution to the problem would be to embark on an intensive program of development of energy derived from an inexhaustible source, such as the sun.

This would establish a new hypothesis, and the process could then move to a new step 2 and work through the process of investigation in a significantly different direction.

The question of nuclear power is obviously only one of an infinite number of problems which can be subjected to scrutiny by the scientific method. For the purpose of our discussion, we can say that many other issues of health and illness have been studied by such scientific analysis. As a result, there are hundreds of specialized areas in which scientific research is going on.

SCIENCE UNDER ATTACK?

An issue which frequently comes to the surface during discussions of health care alternatives is one which is intimately related to scientific investigation. It is sometimes assumed by critics of holistic health care that the scientific method itself is being attacked or ignored during the pursuit of paths other than the traditional Western course of healing. That this view is inaccurate can be seen by looking at but a few of many examples of scientific study in which workers in nontraditional fields are engaged. One of the outstanding examples is the large amount of work which has been done in the rapidly expanding field of biofeedback, both in the United States and in Europe. The work of the Menninger Clinic over the years is well known around the world. Many others have contributed to this literature, including later and less well-known work by C. Maxwell Cade in England, culminating in his recently published work on the development of the "mind mirror."[1] (An excellent article by Anne Bassage later in this book discusses biofeedback further.)

A very extensive body of information has been developed through scientific research into meditation and other altered states of consciousness. One of the largest group of studies has been done by researchers in the Transcendental Meditation program,[2] and other significant contributions have been made by Herbert Benson[3] and many others. A vast amount of scientific literature also has appeared in the fields of holistic nutrition,[4] behavioral kinesiology,[5] radionics, acupuncture,[6] reflexology,[7] iridology and herbal medicine,[8] to mention but a few. Readers of *Body, Mind and Spirit* will become more familiar with some of this literature.

Thus, it becomes very clear that scientific inquiry is very active throughout the various disciplines which make up the holistic spectrum, as indeed it is in all walks of life. Each of us uses parts of the scientific method daily to carry out the simplest tasks. Whenever one builds a greenhouse, or considers a new water system or a composting toilet, many of these steps are gone through.

It has been a pattern of the medical and scientific establishment to label "unscientific" any avenue of inquiry which does not meet rigid standards, especially if the hypothesis is not consistent with the accepted view, and the "bottom line" is not a conclusion provable by objective criteria. A number of examples could be cited, including acupuncture and Oriental medicine in general, still suspect in some quarters while gaining acceptance in others. (The reader's attention is directed to Marc Estrin's fine article on Oriental medicine later in this book.) The same kinds of statements can be made about the attitudes of the traditional establishment toward many of the approaches described or referred to in this book.

WINDS OF CHANGE

One of the bastions of resistance to exploring some of the newer areas in healing has been the American Medical Association (AMA), whose creed is its *Principles of Medical Ethics,*[9] written in 1957. Section 3 of these principles states: "A physician should practice a method of healing founded on a scientific basis; and he should not voluntarily associate professionally with anyone who violates this principle." This has been staunchly defended over the years, and has been the basis for defining certain practitioners, who are not perceived as part of the traditional group, as being unscientific in their work—even, in the eyes of some, as being a threat to the public health. This kind of separation has been made by the currently powerful traditional-practitioner group despite whatever degree of scientific study might be an integral part of the nontraditional discipline under discussion.

It is pleasantly noteworthy that this situation appears to be changing. Since 1977, a special committee of the AMA House of Delegates has been working on a revision of the *Principles of Medical Ethics.* This has not yet been passed, but is currently under study by the component state medical societies. In this proposal, the section quoted above has been deleted, and another proposed section reads: "A physician, except in emergencies, shall be free to choose whom to serve, with whom to associate, and the environment in which to provide service consistent with appropriate patient care."

This proposal will undoubtedly be subject to prolonged and heated debate, with the outcome uncertain, but it certainly appears that organized Western medicine is attempting to move in a direction which will have a liberating effect on its members. The patient population served by the medical profession would surely benefit from the broadening of resources which would be available to them.

MEDICAL HISTORY AT THE FRONTIER

The medical profession in the United States has had an interesting history, and one which is pertinent to any discussion of the present medical model. In the frontier days, there were few medical schools, and those were located mainly in Boston, New York, and Philadelphia. Medicine was a reasonably high art only within a small radius of these cities. Across the vast expanses of the continent, as settlers moved westward, only a trickle of bona fide practitioners went along. In those exacting times, there were undoubtedly as many charlatans and opportunists operating out of the back of wagons, selling flavored river water and diluted whiskey, as there were legitimate health practitioners. As the settlers and their designated warriors ran roughshod over the native Americans, much of the ancient wisdom of the medicine men and women of that culture was stamped out. Very few wise Indian souls survived to pass on that wisdom, and what was passed on was used largely by the native people and not by the white invaders.

This phenomenon of the expurgation of the ancient wisdom has been seen in the history of all the cultures of the world. Western history tells us of Hippocrates, Galen, William Harvey, and Edward Jenner, as well as scores of modern pioneers. But we learn from the oral and written history of all the other cultures that much was known of science and of healing in ancient times which was later suppressed, usually because the possession of such knowledge threatened the dominance of either the church or the state. Much of this ageless wisdom, especially that of the Orient and of native American origin, is being rediscovered today and is becoming part of our expanded knowledge of ourselves and our universe.

MIND AND BODY SEPARATED

Modern medical and scientific thought has been heavily influenced by the French philosopher Descartes (1596–1650), who is generally credited with promulgating the idea that the body and mind are separate entities which can be dealt with in separate ways. This and other later events resulted in the era of specialization in which health care finds itself today. Descartes's theory encouraged separate areas of study to spring up, leading ultimately to heavy emphasis on the treatment of symptoms, syndromes (groups of symptoms), and dysfunctions of physical organ systems.

In the nineteenth century, many events further marked out the course of specialized scientific medicine. The industrial revolution in the Western world, itself a product of advances in scientific knowledge, produced a trend toward urbanization and population growth. In science and medicine, there were a number of developments. Around 1800, Jenner discovered smallpox vaccination. By midcentury, Schleiden and Schwann had proposed the theory that living things were composed of cells. By 1882, Pasteur had found a correlation between microorganisms (germs) and disease, and Koch had discovered the tubercle bacillus. In 1895, Roentgen discovered X-rays, and, by 1900, the Curies had isolated radium. Chemotherapy, the treatment of disease by chemicals, had also begun. Ether and other chemicals were by then in increasing use, thereby facilitating the use of surgical treatment.

THE STIMULUS OF WORLD WAR II

Many of the elements of modern medical practice were thus in place. But the greatest explosion in the medical world was yet to come—World War II. In 1928, Fleming had discovered that the mold penicillin had some effect in the laboratory against germ growth, but the discovery attracted little attention. World War II, more than a decade later, suddenly created a massive need for overcoming infection, and penicillin was rediscovered for the purpose! During that war, there were many other similar examples of accelerated research and expansion of knowledge.

World War II also signaled the greatest economic boom in history, affecting all areas of life. This era of prosperity continued throughout the 1950s. It was during this period that the Western medical establishment became entrenched in a position of unprecedented prosperity and expansion. There were a number of elements in this situation, including a geometric increase in drug production, an explosion in technologic development, a massive infusion of federal revenues into medical and scientific research, and a long-term program of construction and expansion of medical schools.

The Drug Explosion

The enormous growth of the drug industry was unparalleled in history. Old established companies flourished, and new companies quickly became established and grew with remarkable vigor. One factor which is sometimes overlooked is the support given to the drug industry by the petroleum industry. This happened because a large proportion of the drugs undergoing research and in production were petrochemicals, derived directly from the production of other petroleum products, including plastics.

As a result, the market was flooded with scores of new products and formulations, and aggressive personal salesmanship was used to persuade physicians to prescribe the drugs. The most popular drugs were in the classes of tranquilizers, antibiotics, and drugs to lower blood pressure and excrete water. It was not until a number of years after this flood began that the mechanisms designed to control the flow of drugs were tightened up. By that time, both the physicians and the public were quite accustomed to the idea that most diseases were treated by drugs, and that most patients required multiple prescriptions of drugs to maintain a state of health.

Another result of the drug explosion was the gradual recognition of a number of harmful interactions among many of these new drugs, and many hitherto unseen toxic side-effects. Whereas pharmacology had once been merely a basic science, it was now necessary to create a specialty of clinical pharmacology to deal with all of the problems related to the use of prescribed drugs, to say nothing about the burgeoning problem of the illegal use of drugs.

Technological Boom

The explosion of technology ran a course parallel to the drug explosion. The development of the field of cybernetics, including television and computers of increasing complexity, had inevitable effects on what was becoming a health-care industry. One of the effects was the development of high-voltage electron therapy, including cobalt and other therapies widely used in the treatment of cancer patients. There is increasing controversy today about the effectiveness of such therapy relative to its toxic side-effects.

Another effect of the boom in technology is facilitating ever more aggressive and radical surgical approaches in the treatment of disease. Fortunately, this trend is already beginning to subside in some areas, as it has become clearer that the more radical procedures so weakened patients physically and psychologically that their chances for recovery were diminished rather than enhanced.

Federal Aid

The awarding of large and small grants for biomedical research by the federal government of the United States in the late 1940s to the early 1960s had some very significant effects. Firstly, it enhanced the trends in pharmacology and technology described above. In a larger sense, this massive grant program sent a message to the whole scientific world, from Nobel laureates to medical students, that this was where society wanted to put its emphasis for scientific study; this was the wave of the future. The result was great competition among the many specialties in medicine to attract young people to carry on these vast research programs; in effect, to spend the money which was readily available for the asking.

Another important effect of the research explosion was to produce more and more specialization and subspecialization. As a result, the general practitioner nearly became extinct in the United States, until it was finally perceived that the patient was suffering from, among other things, overspecialization. To help correct this situation, "general practice" has been changed to "family practice" and elevated to the status of a specialty, complete with certification, to try to give it a position competitive with the more technical specialties.

The Effect on Cost

The most predictable effect of all the events described here has been a spectacular rise in the cost of health care over the past decade or so. This increase has been above and beyond the general inflation rate, so much so that it probably can be classed as a cause of inflation. There are other causes of the steep rise in costs, among them the increase in malpractice suits, which doctors and hospitals must anticipate in their fees; most authorities attribute this in part to patients' losing confidence in, and closeness to, doctors and hospital personnel. Another cause often referred to is the practice of "defensive medicine" by doctors; that is, if the doctor doesn't order a certain test or procedure, he may be criticized (or sued) by the patient. It is felt that one cause of this predicament is that people expect the available technology to be used. This is called the "technological imperative."

This increase in the cost of health care is causing great concern in government circles because it reflects a grave concern over the general subject of inflation and the threat of recession or depression. Because of this concern, the government is expected to take steps—what steps are uncertain—to halt the rise in health-care costs.

Medical School Expansion

Finally, the construction and expansion of medical schools undertaken after World War II has corrected what was perceived as a doctor shortage. However, as with the sorcerer's apprentice, there seems to be no way to reduce the flow of new doctors now that the "shortage" has been corrected. It is now widely predicted that, by the end of the 1980s, there will be a significant excess of doctors in the United States. This is seen as an unhealthy situation in which competition for available patients can be expected to lead to the performance of unnecessary services. No one can predict at this time how society may wish to deal with this situation.

*   *   *   *   *

In the next chapter, we will look at how cancer, the dread disease of our times, has been thought about and managed over the years. This will shed some light on how our present medical system responds to a strongly challenging situation.

6

Cancer: Symbol and Challenge of Our Time

PETER ALBRIGHT

Nearly 2400 years ago, Hippocrates, the master physician of Greece, taught that illness has natural rather than supernatural causes, and that the human body has the power to heal itself. In that same inspired period in history, the great Essene master teachers passed on the ancient knowledge about proper diet, meditation and healing, which have been reinterpreted for us in the past few decades partly as a result of the discovery of the Dead Sea Scrolls.[1] In this and other ways, the ageless wisdom is being preserved and retold to us in small fragments.

In the 1300s A.D., sixty million people died as the plague swirled across the Old World. Smallpox, and more recently poliomyelitis, have killed and disfigured more. In 1918, twenty million people died as influenza swept the world. It does not seem likely that disease will again bring us devastating scourges of such dramatic dimensions. A little of the great wisdom has been restored to us so that we can immunize against many diseases and "treat" others. Smallpox has now officially disappeared from the globe, and polio's former power is reduced to a mere whimper.

The essential truths about nutrition are just now beginning to be revealed to us. What have appeared to be important advances in this field now give us cause to wonder, and to look further to the natural, whole products of the earth to help us achieve the inner balances we seek.

The "plague" or "pox" of our time is cancer ... Cancer ...

Cancer. The word strikes terror in the hearts of millions (and that is one aspect of it which we all must deal with). Ours is a culture which has to deal in large numbers, and it is very hard not to talk in large numbers when talking about cancer. Millions of words are written about it, millions of dollars are spent in research about it, and millions of dollars are spent in "treating" people who have it each year.

Why talk about cancer in a book about body, mind and spirit? One reason is that so many people *are* so afraid of it. We need to talk a lot about it; if we don't, how can we be creative in our approach to it? Another reason to discuss the subject of cancer is that it encapsulates so much of the thought and action of the western medical model, and shows so much about how people and their problems are dealt with. A further reason to look at cancer is that there is so much happening today to revise our concepts of what cancer is, and how people can deal with it. This chapter, in a way, is only a jumping-off place in this consideration; the rest of the book deals directly or indirectly with how we look at ourselves in relation to the concepts of cancer and other diseases and conditions.

NATURAL HISTORY OF CANCER

What is cancer, then? It is many things. It is a variation on the beautiful story of the growth of human cells—fertilization, the division of cells, the transmission of genetic messages from generation to generation, the eternal seeds of the human race. Growth, like everything else, is a matter of balance. In a system where there is tremendous growth energy, there must be an element which controls the rate of growth, establishes the patterns and sequences, and determines the slowing down and cessation of growth.

In cancer, "something" happens, probably in the element which regulates all these factors of growth, and the character of cell growth and multiplication changes, subtly at first, and then with increasing recklessness. It is the group of factors present at this crucial starting point on which much attention is riveted, both in the "scientific community" and in the minds of many who do not use that label. Of course, that is only the gross starting point, not the real one. The subtler beginnings reside in the subtler realms of the mind, the subconscious, the emotional body, and the spirit. Some people are giving much attention to these areas, and there seems to be a momentum which draws more and more people into this study.

Whatever the impulse or impulses that cause this initial change of course for the cell—and we will talk more of this later—the change does, in fact, occur, either in one spot in the body, or in more than one spot more or less simultaneously. It has long been theorized that the body has relatively little difficulty in reversing this initial change and that, as a regular part of our bodies' health maintenance programs, these microcancers are snuffed out quite frequently, and we are not even conscious that they existed.

Otherwise, after the alteration in cell growth occurs, the cells form colonies of increasing size, eventually becoming appreciable by the physical senses and mechanical aids which we have created for the purpose of sensing. Many of the details of the process are still the subject of theory and observation by scientists in the field. Investigations carried out in the last five years are challenging the traditional hypothesis of tumor spread, which held that the blood stream is of little importance as a route of spread, that tumors spread to regional lymph nodes and through the system in an orderly defined way, and that a tumor is autonomous of its host.

The alternative hypothesis contains a thought which is of great importance to our consideration of cancer: namely, that it is a systemic disease involving a complex spectrum of host-tumor interrelations. Dr. Bernard Fisher has made a number of experimental observations over the past twenty years, summarized in a recent article,[2] which are vital to the newer concepts in tumor biology. If they are generally accepted, the surgical approaches to cancer will continue to be modified to a less radical approach.

EXTERNAL VS. INTERNAL CAUSES

Why does cancer happen? What is behind the "initial" change in cell growth? All the textbooks and encyclopedias virtually up to the present stress mainly two causes, genetics and environment. It is usually stated vaguely that there is probably a "genetic predisposition" to cancer, although there has been clear evidence of this in only one or two kinds of tumor. Then the various environmental factors are discussed which have been linked with cancer in any way—tobacco, excessive sun exposure, viruses, asbestos, soot, etc.—in what might be called the *carcinogen theory*.

Only a few scientists like Fisher, whose work is noted above, are beginning to raise questions about cancer as a systemic disease having roots at deeper levels within the host, rather than a local condition occurring in response to a carcinogen from the outside. On the other hand, other medical practitioners, including Dr. Carl Simonton in the United States and Dr. Ian Pearce in Britain, have arrived by intuition and years of observation and clinical study at the hypothesis that the course of cancer can be influenced by the individual, and that significant causes appear to be rooted in our mental, emotional, and spiritual bodies. Their work and observations will be discussed in later paragraphs. The work of these people and many others is leading us inexorably toward the concept that we can treat patients with cancer in completely different ways, and that healthy people should be treated in some of those same ways in order to maintain healthy balances which, among other things, prevent cancer.

How is cancer treated at present? It is well to have at least a brief look at the conventional way in which people are treated, and at the attitudes behind those methods. First, before cancer strikes, there is the mass programming about the disease, which is clearly a two-edged sword. "Here are the 7 danger signals of cancer" and "Fight cancer with a checkup and a check" are things people have been hearing for years, along with the statistics about death rates from cancer. It can be argued that there is some value to this kind of awareness, but there is increasing doubt as to what that value may be, even the alleged value of periodic physical exams. The negative value is obvious. Worrying about "danger signals" and about the animal experiments showing the carcinogenic effect of the things they eat, drink, breathe, and wear can only lead people to feelings of fear and hopelessness for their future.

STANDARD TREATMENT OF CANCER

The treatment of cancer medically and surgically is becoming an area of increasing public controversy; the illness of young Chad Green of Massachusetts during 1978 and 1979, with the medical and political events surrounding it, is a case in point. As people become more aware and sophisticated about their health, they insist on having more information from their health professionals and a stronger voice in the decision-making process about their own health.

The standard "treatment" of cancer is threefold: surgery, radiation, and/or drugs. Surgery, to state the obvious, is invasive of the body, and it can surely produce deformity, at least at the physical level. This will be discussed further in connection with some emerging concepts in treating cancer of the breast. Radiation has been used for some time as either a primary treatment or in combination with the other methods. Cancer specialists see it as the only way to arrest or slow up some cancers. The theory of radiation is that it affects cancer cells more than it affects normal cells. In practice, it also affects normal cells to some extent, and certain organs are particularly susceptible.

Chemotherapy, or drug therapy, has come into widespread use in cancer in the past twenty-five years, starting with the use of nitrogen mustard, derived from the mustard gas of World War I. There has been a tremendous proliferation of antitumor drugs, and, without exception, they produce serious undesirable side-effects, and can even be fatal. The most serious effects are on the blood-forming organs, especially the bone marrow, and on the immune system, which helps the body fight off bacteria and other offenders when it is in a weakened condition. An all-too-frequent complication of chemotherapy is overwhelming infection.

Even considering all of the untoward effects of standard therapy and the limited gains many patients experience from such therapy, millions of people have received and continue to receive it. It should be clearly acknowledged at the same time that many patients, after receiving standard therapy, are able to resume symptom-free and productive lives; not to state this would be unfair and misleading. The crux of the matter is that, for one reason or another, the standard therapies are not the answer for a significant proportion of people with cancer. If the cancer is too far advanced, or if it is the wrong cell type, or if the patient's general condition is too poor, then too often the message is, "I'm sorry. There's nothing more that can be done."

OPPOSITION TO NEWER METHODS

It is the official position of the cancer establishment today that physicians should not even be exposed to information or ideas originating outside its traditional halls. In a recent incident from this writer's own experience, a distinguished physician was invited to address a state medical convention. The physician had devoted his entire career to the treatment of cancer patients as a specialist in radiology and oncology, and his credentials as a specialist were impeccable. His great genius, and his flaw from the point of view of some of his peers, was that he had gone beyond today's standard therapy. With his deep understanding of human beings and modern physics, he was using, with selected patients, in addition to standard therapy, such modalities as meditation, guided imagery, hypnosis, and intensive counseling. As a result, the patients were feeling better and living longer. But the chapter of the American Cancer Society (ACS) in the state where he was invited to speak, acting on the advice of its oncology consultant, withdrew its support from the physician's appearance on the basis that his practice included techniques which were on the ACS's list of "unproven methods."

One can only hope that such attitudes toward alternative approaches to cancer will soften. The principal objections to the use of alternatives are that they are unscientific, that they may cause delay in the use of standard therapy, and, in some cases, that they may be toxic. The latter argument is interesting in view of what we have said about the toxicity of the standard therapies. On the bright side, one can begin to see an indication of a new trend among physicians which can only lead to better days. This is manifested in a number of ways, perhaps best in the development of the American Holistic Medical Association, a nonprofit organization of "physicians dedicated to medicine of whole person," as it describes itself. The group enrolled over 400 physicians across the United States by the end of its first year, and shows signs of good health and continued growth.

I would like to introduce a few other short stories about cancer which give us cause for cheer and optimism both about the openness of some medical and scientific people to new directions in health and healing and about the sensitivity of some professionals in the late 20th century to the needs and anxieties of people.

CRUSADE AGAINST RADICAL THERAPY

George W. Crile, Jr., has been a distinguished surgeon for many years, working throughout his career at the Cleveland Clinic in Ohio, of which his father was one of the founders. In the mid-

1950s, he became especially interested in the study of cancer of the breast after his wife had contracted the disease. She died of her cancer after having had the entire spectrum of the standard therapy of that time. Dr. Crile launched a study which has now spanned twenty-five years, and which has spearheaded a real change in the attitude of the whole medical profession about the role of radical mastectomy and other therapies for breast cancer. He started by treating small groups of his patients with the less radical therapies, and, as time went on, he was able to demonstrate equally good results to those following radical mastectomy, and, in certain circumstances, even better results.

Thus encouraged, he wrote scientific articles about the results he was achieving, and included more and more patients in his more conservative program. As other surgeons read and heard of his work, they began to try to verify his results. Around the world, in the large cancer treatment centers, the surgeons found that the results were indeed verifiable, and that their patients were managing as well or better than had other patients in identical situations who had been treated by radical mastectomy.[3]

In the spring of 1976, as a result of the accumulation of the results of fifteen to twenty years' experience in all of these centers, the National Cancer Institute in the United States authorized a study comparing the treatment of early breast cancers by three methods other than the radical mastectomy developed by Halsted over eighty years ago and used as the standard treatment ever since. In June 1979, a special report was issued by the National Institutes of Health study group which analyzed the information. The group agreed that a procedure which "preserves the pectoral muscles, i.e., a total mastectomy with axillary dissection, should be recognized as the current standard treatment." What a milestone! The group also agreed that "a diagnostic biopsy specimen should be studied with permanent (slides) before definitive therapeutic alternatives are discussed with the patient." A giant step forward in sharing information with patients! Finally, "The panel supported further clinical investigation into the roles of segmental mastectomy and primary radiotherapy."[4] This is more good news, because segmental mastectomy is a much lesser procedure, and primary radiotherapy implies that, in some cases, no operation may be indicated at all.

Dr. Bernard Fisher, in his editorial comment on this report in the same issue of the *New England Journal of Medicine*,[5] states that the report indicates a better understanding of the biology of tumor spread, lending support to the concept that clinical breast cancer is a systemic disease. The importance of this for all practitioners is enormous, since it depicts cancer as a condition of the entire organism.

THERAPIES COMING CLOSER TOGETHER

This opens up a way to lay to rest the notion that "nothing more can be done." Here we see coming closer together the physician-scientist of the past, who could only make that statement, and the vast assortment of others. Included here are many physicians who have learned from their own experience that "cancer is a condition of the entire organism," and who have been using a number of nontraditional approaches based on the understanding of cancer as a health breakdown on all levels of being—physical, mental, emotional, and spiritual—and finally manifesting on the physical.

A few of these pioneers should be at least briefly mentioned. Dr. Carl Simonton of Texas, working with his wife, Stephanie Matthews-Simonton, and his partner, Dr. Oscar Morphis, has become very well-known for the technique of visual imagery* which he has taught to thousands of his cancer patients, all of whom have already received therapy. Those who receive the special program, which also includes special dietary and counseling instruction as well as the visual imagery technique, are carefully screened to ascertain that they are strongly motivated for their own healing, are willing to work hard in their own behalf, and believe that anything can happen!

Dr. Ian Pearce in England, who has been helping cancer patients for decades, also uses a holistic approach with people who have already had their standard therapy. He sees disease as a loss of balance in a self-balancing system, and cancer as a secondary manifestation of an underlying loss of balance. He has found a number of common items in the emotional histories of cancer patients, and states that a detailed psychological history from childhood is a *must*. His therapeutic regime includes meditation and mental imagery, therapeutic touch, prayer, music, talking in

---

* For discussion of visual imagery, see Chapter 13, "Positive Programs for the Human Mind".

groups over herbal tea, diet management, laetrile in high doses orally, and black coffee enemas for detoxification.

One could cite a number of other practitioners whose patients are experiencing equally good results using a variety of combinations of therapies, but these examples will suffice for the moment. The experience of these practitioners has been that this holistic approach is beneficial to vast numbers of their patients.

It only remains for us now to take that one final difficult step in our thinking, and that is to ask: If this kind of approach is useful to prevent recurrences in patients who have had cancer, why won't it be just as useful to keep people who haven't had cancer from getting it in the first place? It has always been a problem in the field of prevention that you don't know for sure when you have prevented something from happening! In this case, a combination of intuition and experience seems to tell us that changes in consciousness, along with changes in life style, constitute the way to the prevention of cancer, the symbol and challenge of our times.

7

Programming the Human Computer

Body, mind and spirit—all uniquely ours! But, before we are old enough to be aware that the power to be whole comes with this amazing trinity, we are subjected to programming which may make it very difficult to love and accept ourselves as whole beings. We may even have trouble recognizing our true selves by the time our programmers have done with us!

The paradigm changes somewhat over the generations. My mother's programming was largely social and educational. A finishing school taught her to greet inferiors, equals, and superiors in suitable manner. She was sent to schools which taught her the "right behavior" for her position in life. I was programmed for behavior not so much with regard to a social group, but definitely for that appropriate to a *woman.* "Men won't like you if you are too smart," I was told. It was suggested that it was not a good idea to win at tennis too often if you played with a man. I was competitive enough to try to excel in school and to try to win at games, but I felt quite sure that I would be a failure as a result!

PROGRAMMING BEGINS EARLY IN LIFE

Whether our parents are loving and conscientious or callous and indifferent, messages begin to come through very early in our lives.

"Poor child—you are so like me—you've already started to have my headaches." Or "You're the perfect image of your grandfather, and you'll probably come to a bad end just the way he

62

did!" The programming may be more subtle than this, but it finds its way into our thinking and chips away at our wholeness.

If a little boy is impressed by those who care for him that his lot is to play with trucks and tools, that sister's dolls are unsuitable, and that he must not cry over bashed fingers or dead baby birds, then clearly the feminine side of his nature may shrivel up from neglect. If his sister is confined to dolls and toy mops and pans, it may well be difficult for her to develop the masculine side of her nature as she matures. If brother and sister alike are urged to "color inside the lines" in their prestamped coloring books and if they are plopped in front of the TV tube for hours each day, the creative right side of their brains may remain undeveloped.

In addition to negative messages and sex-oriented messages which program the young, there are also garbled messages to add to the confusion. How is the developing psyche to store and sort the information that: Honesty is the best policy, and everyone should be like Honest Abe Lincoln—*but*, when you tell Grandmother honestly that you really have no use for the birthday present she sent you, the adult world descends in wrath and you are disgraced.

Parents are the first programmers. The process begins before birth and continues thereafter. Others soon join the ranks. For some, it might be Sunday school and church where the simple message of Christianity is delivered in totally unrecognizable and useless parcels. How many of us had stamped on our young minds (or was it our knees?) the words, "We have erred and strayed from Thy ways like lost sheep—and there is No Health in us"! What use choking down all that spinach to keep healthy when it is apparently hopeless! Then there is the injunction to "Love thy neighbor as thyself." Clear enough—but neatly contradicted when mother won't let us speak to the lady next door because "She is not a nice person"!

Pretty soon, along comes nursery school, kindergarten, and grade school. School, the seat of learning, about which we have been thoroughly primed ahead of time: It's going to be *such* fun! There we learn not to daydream, more about coloring inside those wonderful lines, and being sure the grass is green and the pumpkin orange—and "Please, Dear, don't cry"! "Sing only when we tell you to, and do not say that something is real when it's only-in-your-imagination."

THE SUPER-PROGRAMMERS

At an early age, the modern child encounters the super-programmers: the media, topped, of course, by television. TV is very real. Mom and Dad watch it, so it surely represents the Truth.

"When you have your next headache," advises the smiling face on the tube, "take something stronger!" Headaches, then, must be a normal part of life.

If your mother doesn't clasp your hand and run through flower-strewn fields with her shiny hair bouncing, just like yours, she is clearly not the right sort of mother. When she is not running, she should be cheerfully supplying you with after-school cupcakes from little cellophane packages and lots of refreshing Kool Aid and wholesome candy and gum. So what's with this bowl of apples and all these nuts and raisins *your* mother keeps handing you?

The growing person, working at self-discovery in this maze of unrealities and contradictions, can, of course, say, "None of this is the way it should be. I will not be fooled or persuaded. I will be strong! I will be *me!*"

But how is a child, an adolescent, or even an adult to make such decisions in a world that is determined to decide for him how he shall feel about himself and his surroundings? And about his future as well?

SOCIAL PROGRAMMING

Social programming is also an important factor, and negative influence in this area is pretty devastating for children growing up as members of minority groups. The black child, native American, or Puerto Rican, has a very tough time coming through the early years with a picture of himself or herself as a powerful, valuable member of the human race whose presence, opinions, and contributions the world eagerly awaits. Even if parents and teachers work overtime to convince such youngsters that they are the light of the world and that they deserve love and support, society is out there shattering this illusion fast.

Children are also frequently prevented by programming from developing into balanced adults with right and left brain functioning strongly. We often ask small children what they want to be "when they grow up," sometimes just to make conversation and sometimes to elicit a cute response. Children usually give a frank and positive answer, and we may laugh and forget it. Then, as the child grows to what we consider a more serious age, we may begin the subtle suggestions of what we determine to be suitable and realistic aims.

The children of today are perhaps less likely to be greatly influenced by their parents' dreams as they choose careers than were children of earlier generations. At the same time, each will be aware of hopes and fears and disappointment, and, even when an honest choice is made, there may be guilt and distress nibbling away at the person who chose a path other than the one the parents hoped for.

There were moments when I thought that perhaps I had not lived up to the expectations of my alma mater as I devoted long years to a concentrated career of child-raising. Such ideas did not help me to feel like a person who had achieved wholeness in the best sense. It was only when I emerged from this stage of my life, when I began to move and grow in new directions with the support and encouragement of my family and friends, that I realized that what really mattered was what I felt about those years, and not what I thought I should feel in relation to others' expectations for me.

THE SCIENTIFIC SCARE PROGRAM

Another sort of programming reaches out to put its message in the computer as we grow into adulthood. It is the scientific scare program. It is valid to point out the possible dangers of carcinogens. But there appears to be a surplus of negative emphasis to the extent that people tend to feel that cancer is lurking in almost everything they touch or enjoy, building up a fear and almost a certainty that we may all develop the dread disease sooner or later. Serious researchers are beginning to suggest that an attitude of negativity, stress, and hopelessness *can* contribute to a predisposition toward developing cancer, so it is important to think about the effects of this kind of programming.

Attempts to sell products such as pain-killers and laxatives and sleep-inducers are often disguised as scientific fact for the not-too-discerning audience by stating that "leading doctors *say*" this or that is highly beneficial. Thus, more misleading information enters the computer.

The amazing thing is that we confidently expect that if we feed and clothe our children decently, keep them clean, take them to the doctor and the dentist, teach them manners, send them to reasonably good schools and colleges, and generally "provide" for them, they will turn out to be polite, well-adjusted, intelligent, presentable, happy, and at least moderately successful. It is always possible that some of them will at least appear to achieve this wonderful combination. However, a great many of us bear into adult life deep scars from the continual programming of our human computers. We need to give careful thought not only to deprogramming ourselves and those who come to us for help, but to preventing the negative and confused programming from ever entering the sacred precincts of body, mind and spirit!

8

The Flowering of the Holistic Era

PETER ALBRIGHT

We have seen how the Western medical model has developed over the centuries, following the expurgation of ancient wisdom in the Middle Ages, into a highly technological industry operating in a complex urbanized society. In this situation, the individual person becomes a minute piece in a gargantuan jigsaw puzzle.

We have traced the thinking through the years about how to manage cancer, and have seen that efforts to contain this disease by logical analytical methods appear to be increasingly frustrating and progressively less productive. This makes us all feel helpless in the face of an "adversary" which our designated experts cannot adequately control.

We have seen how people have devised ways to bring messages to other people, saying that they can expect to be ill with all sorts of diseases—that this is the natural heritage of people—and that, when they become ill, there are multitudes of remedies they can purchase to bring temporary relief.

What we are now coming to realize is that the individual person has the power to remain healthy by becoming whole. We are learning this through rediscovery of ancient wisdom, and through the words of beings now on the planet who, because of the experiences of their past lives or their sensitivity to the natural forces of the universe or their Divine Spark, are in possession of the information which all of us need.

We shall see that, as we pass through all the stages of life on this planet, we can use our Divine gifts and those of our brothers and sisters to find and keep our wholeness, and to restore a healthy state if it slips away from us. We shall see that there are an infinite number of balances in life, which we maintain easily if we know and follow a few simple rules.

The sections which follow are not meant to address each of the situations people face, nor to discuss all of the ways people cope with them. We just have some more friends we would like you to meet who have taught us a lot. We know they will teach you as well, and that you will enjoy them as much as we do.

PART III
Creating and Maintaining Health and Wholeness

9

Sexuality and Well-Being

ANNE COULTER

No account of well-being in our sexual/reproductive function can contain everything there is to know and understand about a subject that has long baffled human beings. Here I present a few reasons why well-being in this aspect of our lives has eluded so many of us, as I have come to understand the reasons, through both my work in family planning and my ponderings about what it means to be a whole person. I also suggest a few reasons for hoping that the confusion and ambivalence which have surrounded our sexuality and our power to create new life need not always be our fate.

MEN AND WOMEN AS PEERS

First, here is a glimpse of how men and women might operate if they had a sense of well-being in this aspect of their lives. Ideally, men and women would regard one another as equals and peers, cheering one another on in their life-long growth toward wholeness. They would feel fully free and able to decide when and if they wished to become parents. They would make sexual intercourse a part of their relationships by mutual and conscious choice only after discussing and agreeing whether or not they wished to become parents at the time. They would take mutual responsibility for contraception if they did not, and then only after discussing and agreeing what they would do should conception occur.

But wouldn't this take all the romance out of it? No, only the nonsense.

CREATORS, NOT VICTIMS

People can and do operate this way, but not as a rule. People are able to do so when they have learned to be creators rather than victims of their experience. Most of us have not been given an opportunity to learn this. We have not been taught the one essential fact of life without which a thorough knowledge of all the other "facts of life" has little meaning. That fact is that human beings are good. Furthermore, we are essentially warm, moral, life-loving creatures, desiring neither to be slaves nor masters, but to grow toward wholeness cooperatively with our fellows.

We humans remain confused and ambivalent about our sexual/reproductive function because we remain confused and ambivalent about our very humanness. We have used the word *human* both to describe what is lovable and noble about ourselves and to explain our weaknesses and failings. We have been very afraid of those weaknesses and failings. The basic fear is that the "dark side" of our nature will overcome the good, destroy our human community, and leave us alone and unprotected in the chaos. In our fear, we have attempted to contain that dark side in ways that have diminished, but not destroyed, the strength and beauty of our essential humanness.

We have, in a sense, created a box to live in, a box which denies that certain facts exist, a box which is about three feet high. Human beings are naturally taller than that. Life at a crouch is painful. We are always striving not only to get out of that painful crouch, but to reach our full height—to become whole. We are like sunflower seedlings that have been planted not in fertile soil in full sun, but in a small box with a hole in one corner of the lid. Like them we grow tangled and matted, competitive, but still we grow, still we reach for the light.

Sunflower seedlings do not have the ability to work together to lift the lid. We do.

In this chapter, the words *health, wholeness,* and *well-being* are used interchangeably. I have come to believe that health, in the World Health Organization's definition, "not merely the absence of disease, but a sense of total physical, mental and social well-being," is all we really want, all we really need, and, appearances to the contrary, is the object of all our strivings. In other words, our struggle may appear to be simply to survive or get out of the crouch. But it is more than that. Our struggle is to become whole human beings.

Reared in a dark, cramped box where our humanness is not encouraged to flourish, the ways we strive to reach wholeness are sometimes hurtful to ourselves and others. This serves to perpetuate and rigidify our fear of that dark side. Never are we collectively so insecure and afraid as in times when the human spirit, as it always will, comes shining through in spite of it all and threatens to change things by punching more holes in the lid of our safe little box to let in the light.

BIRTH CONTROL AND SEXUALITY EDUCATION

One such time was 1917, when Margaret Sanger began her crusade to challenge the anti-vice Comstock Laws and to bring birth control information to American families. Another beam of light was the publication of Albert Kinsey's work in the late forties and early fifties.[1] (At the time, I was a young, box-reared teenager. My friends and I were eagerly sending away for free booklets on the "facts of life" to be mailed to us in "plain brown wrappers." But I can remember thinking there was something a little nasty about Dr. Kinsey's preoccupation with sex.)

In our own time, the movement for more holistic sexuality education and the movement for women's liberation have made the box feel less secure for many of us. But both are profoundly humanistic movements. They hold promise for removing some of the barriers to a humane, integrated understanding of our sexual/reproductive selves and to making decisions about this aspect of our lives which proceed from a sense of wholeness.

When the subject of "sex education" comes up, there are as many reactions as there are people in the room. These reactions often spring from unexamined fears. To one, sex education holds the threat of providing information to the young that would be like providing them with burglar's tools. To another, it might mean relief from instructing his own children in "such a difficult matter." Our fears, not our cussedness, have kept us from agreeing what sex education should be, who should do it, when, and for whom. So, as a rule, we have done nothing. And the young have inherited our fears, our ignorance, and our ambivalence.

This inheritance has produced a fractured, piecemeal under-standing of reproductive health and sexuality and has meant that many human beings have had to learn by bitter experience how all-of-a-piece it is with our total well-being.

Once, while sitting in a friend's kitchen, I noticed an emphatic memo on the family bulletin board, "Feed Jacques comfrey every day!" It was the stud season of my friend's prize goat. The com-frey was intended to insure his vigor and that of his offspring. I was new to the field of family planning at the time and dismayed that so many people seemed to understand the words "family planning" and "reproductive health" as euphemisms for having sex without having babies. I wondered wistfully how long it would be before we humans come to understand family planning as a matter of health care, as did my friend the goatkeeper.

Talking with patients at our family-planning center, I usually ask if they have had an opportunity to learn how their reproduc-tive systems work and how conception takes place. The most common response is, "Not really." The next most common re-sponse is, "Well, a nurse came and showed us a movie in the (fourth, sixth, or eighth) grade." Studies of pregnant teens in this country underscore their ignorance about human fertility, but ig-norance alone is not responsible for what has been called the epi-demic of teenage pregnancy in the United States. Reproductive plumbing lessons alone are not the answer to our tragically poor preparation for our reproductive years, nor do they teach us what we want and need to know to live in health with our sexuality and reproductive powers. Neither does the laying on of dire warnings and moral preachments, which has been such a rich part of our heritage.

Whether we are victims or creators of our experience in any as-pect of our lives depends not only on what we learn, but on how we learn it. We begin learning about our sexuality and human re-lationships the moment we are born, and all that we learn be-comes part of ourselves. The question is: shall we be able to look in a mirror and see ourselves clearly in relation to what we have learned? Or is the mirror cracked and broken, offering back a fractured, disconnected reflection of ourselves?

In the past ten years, we have begun to see that sexuality edu-cation is already happening and that our task is to help the young integrate it into their total experience. Church bodies (The United

Methodist, United Presbyterian, and Unitarian, for example) have undertaken family-oriented, human-sexuality education projects. There has been a profusion of books written for parents, teachers, and for the young themselves. Most exciting, perhaps, is the growing number of public-school districts that are grappling with the issue. Although they have often been motivated by alarm over teen pregnancy rates, they are, nevertheless, overcoming the paralysis of fear that has kept us from action on this "dark" subject for so long. A number of large school districts in various parts of the country have involved teachers, parents, and students in the agonizing, but very democratic process of defining what sexuality education should be, and how and by whom and for whom it is to be taught. What they have come up with is an understanding that it must begin early and that it must not be taught as a subject apart, but within the context of understanding and controlling one's health and well-being. And, this, of course, includes learning about human relationships, feelings, and emotions as well as about our wonderful ears and lungs. It includes, as well, exploring what it means to be male or female right now, and critically examining our assumptions about maleness and femaleness.

An important realization we are making about sexuality education, wherever it takes place, is that learning must include and build on the profound human need, seen most unabashedly in small children, to process, question, make sense of our day-to-day experience with our peers. This means that adults do not deliver information so much as they help young people help each other discover and believe in their self-worth and ability to make good decisions about their lives.

To illustrate: Most children learn a great deal from the mass media, a great deal that goes unprocessed. One of the things that has been learned too often without getting processed, and therefore is accepted as fact, is an understanding of sex as an "uncontrollable urge." Rarely does the sexual coming together of men and women in the movies or on television seem to have anything to do with creating babies.

The staff members of our family-planning center are often asked to talk to high-school classes about contraception. This we do, if it rounds out or is part of a whole learning experience for the students. That is, we do it if we are not there only to inflict on them contraceptive information out of context. In classes where a feeling of safety for discussion already exists, I have sometimes asked students to consider how we would understand and make decisions about our sexuality and human relationships if all we knew was what we had learned from advertisements, movies, television, and the lyrics of popular songs. I have seen students come to a very good understanding of why contraception would not be used or even discussed by men and women if this were so. And they have contributed example after example of how the myth of the "uncontrollable urge," I-can't-live-without-you-baby, is perpetuated in the mass media—and the myth generally explodes in their healthy laughter. An adult cannot guide young people through the sexual mythology that abounds in our world in a useful and helpful way merely by talking at them. Young people must be involved in this process.

SEXUAL MYTHOLOGY

The movies, television, and popular songs are not responsible for creating this sexual mythology, nor are they entirely responsible for its perpetuation. They merely reflect the fact that we often unconsciously seek to find completeness, or a missing sense of wholeness, through sexual activity. This has made sex and being sexually attractive such a preoccupation in our society. If we can understand this, we can begin to understand a bit better why the connection between our sexuality and our fertility is so often unconsciously denied, and why, as a result, there are so many unwanted children in this world.

THE WOMEN'S MOVEMENT

One of the reasons for our sense of incompleteness is the greatly troubling and unhealthy dependence of men upon women, and women upon men. This dependence has been the fruit of the institutionalized inequality of men and women. It is this situation that the historical women's movement, powerfully reemerged in the last ten years, would change. It is a movement that would profoundly change our lives. It would not destroy our human community and its cornerstone, the family, as some fear, but, in fact, would strengthen both. It is not the work of nasty, deviant, "unfeminine" women. It is the human spirit shining through, as it always will, to bring light into darkness.

Periods of change are not particularly comfortable times. Like Pandora's box, they do, indeed, unleash demons. The demons are all our unexamined fears flying around frantically in the unaccustomed light.

By talking with one another and writing for one another, women have examined and shown one another what their experience has been. They have given one another the courage to be victims of it no longer. They have helped one another understand and take charge of their own bodies and health—to disclaim the narrow view of women's psychology, essential nature, and work in this world. They have helped one another to have a clear vision of themselves as strong, intelligent creatures, no longer to be dominated and defined by men, but to be their peers and equals. A sharing, rather than a reversal, of roles is envisioned. The women's movement is a profound rejection of the view of women as the only nurturers of society, functioning primarily in the home. It is a clear statement that the work of nurturing human beings so that they may be whole is the work of both sexes all of the time in any activity that touches human lives.

Men have felt uncomfortable in the nurturing role not because it goes against their essential nature, but because this deeply human capacity has been seen as a female trait and has not been encouraged in men. What has been encouraged in men is strength, aggressiveness, decisiveness, and suppression of feelings and emotions. Often, in life's extremity, such as in combat, men have learned about their ability to express feelings and fears and to support and physically comfort one another. In regular life, it does not seem safe to do so. In the pain of crouching around in the box, men have turned not to each other, but to women for comfort. And women who have learned to measure their worth by their attractiveness to men have bought into this. This unhealthy, unexamined dependency between men and women has been one of the major reasons why male-female relationships are so often fraught with anger, anxiety, noncommunication, and sexual irresponsibility.

Most men have not greeted the women's movement with gladness. It is not easy to accept the fact that one has been an oppressor, and, at the same time, to hang on to one's feeling of self-worth. Yet, more and more (not yet enough, but more) men have begun to see that the changes envisioned by the women's movement threaten to destroy nothing more than what has kept men and women from being fully human. Men have begun to examine their lives and experiences and to write about it for one another. They have begun to want to share the decisions involved in conception and contraception and in the process of birthing and nurturing their children.

Things are changing. We ought not to deny it, but to acknowledge it and to talk about it deeply with one another—and with our young.

A glimpse was offered above of how men and women might function if they had a sense of health and wholeness about their sexuality and reproductive powers. Implicit in that glimpse was the ability to communicate with other human beings and to make decisions consciously and without distress. I have tried to point to some of the things that have kept us from making conscious decisions that proceed from a sense of wholeness.

TO BE—OR NOT TO BE—PARENTS

One of the conscious decisions we should be encouraged to make is whether or not we want to become parents. The couple who wishes to remain childless has been regarded as unfortunate or misguided. Suspicion has been widespread that people who do not have children are incomplete. Now, there seems to be growing understanding that this need not be so. There is even an organization called The National Organization for Optional Parenthood, which exists to make the statement that it is important for people to decide whether they really want to become parents.* Is it not? The importance to our sense of well-being of making decisions surrounding conception and contraception cannot be exaggerated.

If a couple has decided to be sexually active and has decided not to conceive, each must also decide how important it is not to conceive. This will influence their decision about how to contracept. They must decide whether the possible immediate or long-term risks to the woman's health and fertility involved in the use of oral contraceptives or the IUD are acceptable. If they choose a statisti-

* National Organization for Optional Parenthood, 3 North Liberty Street, Baltimore, Maryland 21201.

cally less reliable method, they must decide if they are willing to abstain from intercourse before and during the woman's fertile period or to use another method at this time. And, because all methods of birth control presently available can fail, they must also decide what they would do should conception occur despite their best efforts.

NATURAL BIRTH CONTROL

Perhaps because ever growing numbers of people are consciously seeking to live holistically, there has been a noticeable increase of interest in natural methods of birth control. One of these, a more scientific version of the rhythm methods, is being actively promoted and taught by Catholic and nonsectarian groups here and throughout the world. Generally called the sympto-thermal method, the process involves the woman's daily monitoring and charting of her basal body temperature and cervical mucus, both indicators of the time of ovulation. Used in its purest form, the method involves abstinence from intercourse prior to and during a woman's fertile period. The method involves a great deal of education, and, as can be imagined, a great deal of understanding and ability to communicate well among those who practice it. It has been a highly successful method for some people, both practically and spiritually. But the method, for all the beauty of its naturalness and wholeness, is not fail-safe. Even so, natural methods of birth control will probably grow in popularity as men and women move more consciously toward wholeness by sharing in the planning, birthing, and nurturing of their children.

Natural methods will never meet the needs of all people. It is not appropriate for those who are in the process of deciding whether or not they ever wish to be responsible for creating another human life nor those for whom a conception would be a far greater risk than one associated with a reliable chemical or mechanical method of birth control.

FUNDING FOR BIRTH CONTROL

People who come to our family-planning center often ask about new methods of birth control that are in the experimental stage. We have to tell them a fact of life about which many are unaware.

That is, that although there are many ideas for better methods of contraception, public funding for research and the expensive clinical trials mandated by the FDA are woefully inadequate. This was the conclusion of a two-year Ford Foundation study, "Reproduction and Human Welfare," published in 1976 involving 200 scientists. They stated that by 1980 we should be spending $500 million annually on contraceptive research and development, or about three times as much as we now spend. As a colleague of mine recently pointed out, "We spend as much for one B-1 bomber as we do for contraceptive research in one year." This is another opportunity for the human spirit to punch more holes in the lid of our box.

Our search for health and wholeness in conception and contraception must proceed in several ways. One is, surely, to commit ourselves to improving the choices people have in contraceptive methods. Another is a commitment to examine and root out the fear that has kept us from being whole in this important aspect of our lives and that has prevented us from realizing and celebrating our wonderful humanness.

10

Birth: A Unifying Experience

PAT SWARTZ

Birth is one of the major emotional and physical experiences of human life. As such, it unites us all with a common bond no matter what social, economic, educational, or racial background we may have. No one can be closely involved in a birth experience without being in some way affected by it. It is a sudden and awesome confrontation with ourselves as living things. Birth changes our role from being solely someone's child to being parents of a new generation, and, in so doing, puts new demands upon our strengths and weaknesses.

There is a close relationship between society and birth. The attitude of our society towards birth mirrors the attitude of many of its members towards life in general. Since the advent of medical technology, this attitude has been somewhat like that of a spectator, isolated and protected from the rigors of the game of life. By choosing to stay on the periphery only, we may, as a result, extract little excitement and fulfillment from the true business of living. The past decade has seen gradual and welcome changes. More and more people are feeling the need to take control over their lives and to participate actively in the natural experiences which life offers.

BIRTH: POSITIVE AND NEGATIVE

Birth, as an experience of life, can be both positive and negative. As a positive experience, it can be exciting, fulfilling, awe-inspiring, and delightful. It can be a unifying experience, enriching a person's self-esteem, strengthening family ties, and generating strong maternal and paternal feelings. This, in turn, gives to society strong family units of caring individuals with a desire for total involvement with life and well-developed feelings of personal responsibility.

Birth as a negative experience can be destructive to society. As a frightening, painful, humiliating experience it causes alienation and grief. These feelings result in a poor self-image for the woman and feelings of guilt in her male partner. These feelings may in turn be reflected in disturbed family relationships. Under these circumstances, it is more difficult for good maternal and infant bonding to occur, which can lead to poorly developed family ties and even abusive relationships.

Assuming our ultimate goal to be that of total involvement with life and the assumption of responsibility for our health and well-being, we may take birth as a good starting point. The prenatal period is a great time for a woman to begin taking charge of her health and the health of her unborn child. In order for birth to be the most positive experience possible, we must consider some necessary ingredients.

BIRTH AS A NORMAL PROCESS

Most people would probably say that one of the most important ingredients for a positive birth experience is good health. I include here both physical and mental health and some things which contribute to these. The basic starting point is the acceptance of birth as a normal, natural process of the body rather than a disease. This acceptance has to be shared by both the parent-to-be and her doctor. Many doctors, even in present times, see birth as a situation of disease. This is, in great part, a result of their training, usually in large medical centers where a larger than normal proportion of the maternity patients are "high risk" patients or patients with special problems. It is crucial for a doctor in training to learn how to handle all unusual and dangerous situations and to gain expertise with sophisticated equipment for treating such cases. However, the outcome is that many newly qualified doctors are more aware of the problem situations than of the normal birth process. It is difficult for such a doctor to relate to a patient who is asking for a noninterventionist approach to her child's birth. Both patient and doctor must be prepared to invest time in trying to understand the other's point of view. From this, a relationship based on trust can evolve.

This feeling of trust in her doctor does not mean that the patient is abdicating her responsibility for her own health care. It is the basis of an important partnership working toward a healthy positive pregnancy and birth. Forming such a relationship is not always easy, especially for the very young woman or the one who feels threatened by all figures of authority. In such situations, it is important for the doctor to try to initiate a trusting relationship. Sometimes, it may seem easier and quicker to adopt an attitude of paternalism (or maternalism) and assume the total decision-making role. This does not help the patient to grow emotionally and merely fosters her original feelings of powerlessness.

In many ways, our society tends to emphasize the negative aspects and complications of pregnancy and birth rather than the basically healthy state. Morning sickness, constipation, and hemorrhoids all receive more attention from friends and relatives than the glowing aura of a contentedly pregnant woman. No one would deny the existence of these discomforts of pregnancy, but, to a great extent, they can be minimized by a good diet, exercise, and involvement of body and mind in activities which distract the person from self-centered concern.

PHYSICAL CHANGES IN PREGNANCY

Pregnancy is a time of heightened awareness of the body and its functions. In fact, it may be the first time that some women become aware of the uncontrolled forces of a living body at work. Most of us are quite familiar with our external appearance, but few of us frequently think about our insides. During pregnancy, it is impossible to ignore changes in shape and proportion of the body, skin and hair changes, and fluid retention. During pregnancy, a woman may, for the first time, really become familiar with the location and activity of such organs as the bladder, lungs, stomach, and, of course, the uterus. It is important to understand what is happening inside the body in order to relate to the activities and sensations of these organs. With such knowledge, steps can be taken to help the body function more smoothly.

Most of the physical changes of pregnancy are related to and controlled by hormonal changes or changes in the body chemistry. Many of these changes, both physical and chemical, result in emotional changes which, if not appreciated, may be a source of concern. Heightened sensitivity may cause temper flare-ups, tears for no apparent reason, irrational fears, ambivalence toward both partner and baby, and undesirable feelings of dependence and depression. It is important for a happy pregnancy and an emotionally healthy birth experience that a woman recognize her emotional swings, realize their origins, and talk about her feelings and concerns with an understanding person. Once again, physical and mental activity with other people prevents brooding on fears and helps stimulate good mental health.

PREGNANCY AND NUTRITION

Good health of body and mind are dependent on good nutrition, rest, and exercise.

In the case of a planned pregnancy, there is no excuse for becoming pregnant while not in optimum health. Many studies have shown that good health and nutrition of both parents are important to the achievement of a baby with the highest possible mental capacity. It is ironic that, unlike most farmers, who take special care to prepare their stock for future breeding, many human parents are very inadequately prepared in terms of nutritional needs. It is frequently stated that the fetus will take what it requires for growth from the mother's body. Though this is true, it is a very casual, offhand way to describe fetal nutrition and the devastating effects this may have on the mother, the baby, and future generations.

The old adage about the need to eat for two during pregnancy may not be so far from the truth. This doesn't necessarily mean the quantity of food eaten, but the quality and nutritional balance of the diet. When a woman becomes pregnant, she is often ready to make a commitment to better eating habits "for the sake of the baby." It is essential that those supporting this woman, her family, partner, doctor, and friends, encourage her to improve her diet and give up harmful habits involving drugs, alcohol, and tobacco.

Physicians have a duty to inform their patients of the importance of good nutrition and to take the time to make sure that *all* their patients understand what this means. Many studies have shown that poor nutritional habits in America cut across all socio-economic levels. Physicians cannot assume that any patient has an adequate diet unless they take the time to find out.

"Eating for two," in the positive sense of the phrase, means finding out what the body requires to provide the best sources of energy and raw materials not only for the growth and development of the baby, but also for the growth, development, and healthy maintenance of the mother's body during pregnancy. This includes providing for healthy development of the placenta, the formation of the expanded blood volume, the growth of breast tissue and uterine muscle, and the provision of energy for the increased activity of heart, lungs, and kidneys. Vitamins and iron supplements do not provide all these raw materials, and yet these continue to be the main thrust of the nutritional component in many prenatal care programs.

Good nutritional habits acquired during early pregnancy, combined with good support and encouragement, can have an added bonus: if maintained after the birth of the baby, they provide a firm foundation for the health of the new family.

EXERCISE AND PREGNANCY

The changes of pregnancy are vigorous and many. They are enormously energy-consuming. To many women, one of the first signs of pregnancy is a feeling of sleepiness or general fatigue. Part of the awakening consciousness of the body is the awareness of changes such as this unusual tired feeling. Some women will try to ignore such feelings, others will give in and take more naps. It is important to recognize such feelings and to try to supply the body's demands. Early pregnancy is a time of upheaval and re-orientation of the body's physiology towards new biological needs. Late pregnancy is a time for the body to prepare physically for the huge energy consumption of birth. The need for rest at both ends of the pregnancy should be met so that the body may function more efficiently.

Some women are afraid of exercise during pregnancy. They sit around, becoming bored and dwelling on fears and minor physical problems, and, in general, becoming very self-centered. This inactivity also has other undesirable effects. Poor circulation, sluggish bowel activity, a tendency to poor posture and back trouble, all can result from lack of exercise. Unless medically indicated otherwise, exercise and pregnancy go well together. Most physical activities which have been done before pregnancy can be continued, though sometimes less strenuously. Brisk walking is an excellent form of exercise for those who are not the athletic type. Most childbirth preparation courses include some physical exercises which are specially designed for added comfort during the last part of the pregnancy. Exercising the body creates a sense of well-being and instills confidence. It helps a woman to feel more in charge of her body rather than as a prisoner in an expanding, fleshy blob. This leads to a more confident outlook on birth itself.

SUPPORTIVE MEDICAL CARE

Since the human body is not a machine, and since all bodies do not function equally well even given optimum conditions, it is important that all pregnant women receive good supportive medical care. This care is geared towards the most positive outcome of birth we can hope for—a healthy mother and child. I have already mentioned the establishment of a trusting, working partnership between patient and doctor. Some women tend to forget that they are paying their doctor for the care they receive. They are, in fact, employing this health-care professional to help them achieve a healthy and happy experience. If they do not intend to use his expertise and advice, they should not employ him, but should find another doctor with whom they feel more comfortable. By the same token, the doctor should not forget who is having the baby and what his patient's real needs are. One of the greatest things a doctor gives to a patient is *time*. This is what supportive medical care is all about. To a woman having a normal, healthy pregnancy, one of her doctor's finest qualities is being willing to take time to answer her questions. Unwillingness of medical professionals to invest time in emotional support of their patients has encouraged many women in recent years to seek alternatives to doctor-attended hospital births. Women must be given the information needed and the opportunity to make choices and decisions about their birth experiences and their prenatal care.

No pregnant woman should assume that her body will perform as she wants it to without having had a doctor's opinion on the subject. Our bodies are complex and many things about them are hidden from us. A woman needs to know that her body is tolerating pregnancy well, that the baby is developing properly, and that the baby has a good chance of getting out of her body without trouble. These things cannot be assumed no matter how fit she feels, and, for these reasons, no woman should reject medical care during pregnancy.

SUPPORT FROM FAMILY AND FRIENDS

Support comes not only from the doctor or midwife, but also from the woman's partner, her extended family, and her friends. I have already mentioned some aspects of support concerning good nutrition and health habits. There must also be support for the new young parents by the older generation. Their choice of medical personnel, location of birth, and method of birth are all movements towards the assumption of new roles in life with new personal responsibilities. Understanding parents will help their children make their own decisions about these things and will support their choices, though these choices may not be the directions which they themselves would have taken. This type of support is very important to a young, single mother who may find her role difficult to assume, especially if she is either over-protected or totally rejected by her extended family.

The woman's partner, also, must try to understand the physical and emotional changes of her body and appreciate the strains which these place upon her. Giving his support and concern in preparing for labor, and during labor and birth itself, can enhance the relationship and strengthen the emotional bonds of the couple. A new nursing mother may need a lot of support and encouragement from her partner, family, and friends until she gains self-confidence and skill. It is so important to build early confidence in parenting skills that those who deal with new parents should do all they can to provide the needed support.

CHILDBIRTH PREPARATION CLASSES

One way in which both parents can come to understand the changes of pregnancy and the process of birth is through childbirth-preparation classes. Classes are now provided in many com-

munities as parents have demanded more preparation and knowledge than they were able to obtain elsewhere. The classes vary in
content from those stressing baby care and the post-partum period to those providing exercises for pregnancy and techniques for
labor and delivery.

The popularity of childbirth preparation has grown as more
knowledge has been acquired and popularized about the negative
effects on the baby of medications given to the laboring woman.
The popular press and other media have also stimulated interest
in prepared childbirth. The fear of losing control under the influence of medication has encouraged many women to participate
more fully in the birth process. The positive, joyful experiences of
so many prepared couples is the best form of advertising and has
led to almost total acceptance of the classes as an integral part of
the prenatal period.

Though preparation for childbirth does not rule out the use of
drugs, it does minimize their use in normal labor and delivery. It
also allows a woman, through control and relaxation, to cooperate
more fully with her doctor, making the labor and delivery easier
and pleasanter for all involved. Though termed by many "natural
childbirth," the techniques are actually learned or conditioned responses to labor and not "natural" at all.

Several methods of birth preparation are available in America
today, all of them involving breathing and relaxation or muscular-
control techniques. The basic goals of all the methods are to help
the body work more efficiently by conserving energy through
conscious muscular relaxation and by providing an adequate oxygen supply to the uterine muscles. The breathing patterns which
supply the oxygen are, in some methods, also used as a mental
barrier preventing the brain from perceiving stimuli from the
uterus, normally perceived as pain.

Along with the techniques for labor and delivery, the classes
include a lot of factual information about physiology, anatomy,
and the process and sensations of labor. This information breaks
the fear-tension-pain cycle which normally provides a barrier to a
pleasant labor. The involvement of the baby's father or another
supportive person in the classes and in labor and delivery is a valuable and integral part of the preparation process and enhances
emotional ties between family members.

Related to the childbirth classes are two important incidentals.

First, the classes themselves provide an additional support system for the new parents, giving them a place to share feelings and concerns with others in the same stage of pregnancy. Secondly, the classes provide a source of consumer information on hospital practices and policies and community services for parents and infants. This informed consumerism can be a powerful source of positive change in the delivery of medical services to young families.

THE LOCATION

Through informed consumerism, young parents have a much better chance of selecting the location for their birth experience best suited to their needs and desires. When planning for the best possible experience, it is important to select the location with the most positive features. For a hospital birth, find a hospital with the best medical options in case of emergency, one where each patient is treated as an individual and not given routine treatment whether or not it is needed. The staff should be supportive, ready to answer questions, and ready to coach breathing techniques if necessary. Flexibility within the system is important when planning such options as the position for the delivery, the location of the delivery, such as birthing room, labor room, or delivery room, and the arrangements for early contact with the baby and early breast-feeding. All these options should be worked out in advance of labor with the doctor, and, if necessary, with the hospital, so that birth itself can flow smoothly without concern for logistics.

THE CESAREAN BIRTH

In the preparations so far, we have assumed that the birth will go as planned with no major problems. This is what we all hope for, but, as we know, it is not what always happens. All pregnant women should confront some of the negative alternatives to a straightforward birth. One of these alternatives is Cesarean birth, which has become more frequent in recent years.

There are many reasons for this increase, but the two most significant are the improvement in safety of the technique and early warning of fetal distress caused by continuous electronic fetal monitoring. It is not my purpose to discuss whether or not the rise in the Cesarean rate is justified, but to remind women that this is a method of birth for which they should all be prepared. Those women who are prepared for the Cesarean birth-experience, whether planned or unexpected, have a more positive experience and a more speedy recovery. Since many hospitals are now allowing fathers to attend Cesarean births, it is also very important that they are also prepared. The presence of the father in the operating room gives him yet another opportunity to support his partner, with added insight, through the surgery and recovery period.

In all births, the presence of both parents in cases of extreme fetal distress or death contributes to their mutual support through the grieving process. Excluding one parent only adds to the stress on both of them when confronting complications.

THE POSTPARTUM PERIOD

Planning a positive birth also includes planning for the early postpartum period. Recent trends in postnatal care have shown concern for the gentle handling of the newborn infant in the period immediately after birth. Those parents concerned and interested in applying the so-called Leboyer Method will want to make sure, in advance, that both their physician and hospital are familiar with and supportive of their wishes. Recent work in the field of maternal and infant bonding has revealed its far-reaching effects on the development of maternal behavior and has highlighted the need for parents and infant to remain in close contact immediately after birth. Again, this is a facet of the birth experience to be planned for in advance. Breast-feeding immediately after delivery and rooming-in with sibling visitation allow all to contribute to a positive family birth experience and are becoming more widely available.

THE BIRTHING ROOM

With the institution of the birthing-room concept, birth in the hospital can truly be a family experience. The birthing-room concept is an outgrowth of pioneer work by the Maternity Center Association of New York in out-of-hospital birthing centers. Birthing rooms are a means of providing a home-like setting for birth at low cost but with the safety features of hospital delivery close at hand for emergency use. Patients are carefully screened, and only those with no apparent or foreseen health problems are encouraged to use the birthing center or birthing room. The patient usually requests the minimum of intervention and medication unless it becomes necessary to use these tools. Labor and delivery take place within the same bed in the same room, and other family members, including children, may be present at the discretion of the physician. After a short recovery period, usually of twelve hours, the mother and baby are discharged with follow-up provided by community nursing services.

This type of birth experience combined with the preparation outlined above is a wonderful way of expanding the awareness of healthy body-function in all family members. New, improved eating and sleeping habits, exercise, and general knowledge can be forged into attitudes of personal responsibility for health which will last for a lifetime.

In modern times, when many families are planned in advance and the number of children in a family is small, it is especially important that each birth be a positive experience. This great life process with all its powerful potential is too valuable to be left to chance.

11

Moving through Life and Dealing with Hurts

STEPHEN PARKER AND SUSANNE TERRY

Between birth and the state that we term *adulthood* is an extended period called *growing up*. This consists, in part, of achieving physical maturity—mastery of the muscular system, developing strength, coordination, and agility—as well as collecting large amounts of understandable information and shrinking the areas that are unknown.

THE GROWING-UP PROCESS

The growing-up process is far from fully understood, and there are many common misconceptions about it. For example, for a long time, a notion was prevalent among doctors and nurses that babies really were not aware of what was happening to them at birth. The result of this thinking was the use of bright lights, cold forceps, and rough treatment in the delivery room. Dr. Leboyer, in his book *Birth Without Violence*,[1] has made it clear that this thinking is not valid. He felt that this misconception was based upon the blocking out by adults of the painful memories of their own birth experience. In recent times, many people have uncovered real and agonizing memories of their own birth. It is apparent that the experience of birth leaves a profound imprint for better or worse upon the individual's character.

The rigid structure of our society has kept us from understanding well how children function. The needs of society have dictated the place we give to children. This has certainly not always been in their best interests. There was, for example, a time when there was virtually no such thing as childhood as we now think of it, because of the society's work and economic needs. Children at five and six were often expected to have responsibility for younger children, and then, at seven or eight, they were expected to learn a trade.

Today, childhood is prolonged and extended. During a short period in children's lives, they are viewed romantically by adults. They are surrounded with adoration, dressed in carefully selected clothing, and cameras record every move and every stage of progress. (Dewy-eyed adults are caught up in the mystery and beauty of childhood.) Many families, of course, cannot afford the time or money required to create a romantic aura around childhood, but they cannot escape the idea that this is the way they "ought" to be relating to their children, if only they had not suffered the misfortune of poverty.

At some point, adults begin to leave the romanticized notions behind and start worrying about whether the child will develop in an acceptable manner. Most of us were burdened as children with the feeling that adults were more concerned about how we would turn out than about who we really were at any given time.

This frustration intensifies during the teenage years and often escalates to the desperate cry, "You don't care about me at all! All you care about is your own reputation and what people will think." That is not entirely true, of course. But the young person has correctly perceived that he is often not fully appreciated by the parent. Instead, what is being expressed to the child is worry and concern about the future.

If a common societal view of children is marked either by romanticism or worry about the end product, what does this say about our perception of what children are really like? One need only try to wade through the morass of books, pamphlets, schools of thought, and popular theories about children to see that there have been many attempts to understand early childhood. It is very difficult, however, to know where to find accurate information about the nature of young humans! Our own experiences as children and with children result in many conflicting statements that make it difficult to generalize. There are, however, certain statements that we can safely make after reflecting carefully on our own childhood and by observing children.

These statements are: first, that children are born whole and with natural intelligence; second, that children are repeatedly hurt in their growth processes; third, that they have a natural mechanism for healing the hurt; and fourth, that this mechanism is often interrupted, causing the hurt to be retained.

Let's look more carefully at these statements in terms of what we have observed.

First, children are born whole, with intelligence and flexibility. They spend many years in a constant learning process to develop thought processes, vocabulary, sophisticated logic systems, uses of motor skills, and other necessary abilities. Children are eager to learn and naturally assume that the world is a safe place for them. They are able to master complicated tasks quickly and are involved in an ongoing process of learning about their environment. What children do not have to learn is their own emotional healing process.

A MECHANISM FOR HEALING HURTS

We have also stated that children have a mechanism of their own for healing the hurts that come to them in their growing process. Unfortunately, we often interrupt this healing process before it is completed, causing the hurt to be retained as the source for later trouble.

What happens if you startle a baby? He jumps. He might cry—and will cry as long as he wants to, regardless of your need to talk on the telephone or your desire to watch television. If you forget to feed the hungry child, she will remind you in no uncertain terms. If a toddler stumbles and is hurt, he will announce it clearly. If a door won't open or a jar come unscrewed, howls of anger will resound through the neighborhood. A child will not tolerate hurt; there is an immediate reaction. She may be screaming, crying, sniffling, or shaking. This will continue until we feel it will never stop—and then, suddenly, it stops, and the child returns to her stack of toys and begins playing again. Healing has taken place.

As adults, we have a difficult time letting children continue their healing process as long as they want to. We storm, "Enough is enough!", "I'll give you something to cry about," or, "I've got things to do, and I can't have this." Because it is hard for us to take, or because we do not have enough help in dealing with it properly, we find ways to stop "all the fuss." But the "fuss" is what heals, and we haven't let it quite finish.

The result of our impatience is that the hurt is retained. No one ever loses information. When the child's need to release in his own way is interrupted, the experience is recorded. Somewhere in the information system of the young person is something which says, "This is a hurtful experience."

The ways in which we are hurt cause certain protective behavior. The child may become more shy or more belligerent in an attempt to protect himself from further hurt. Remember looking at the young, relatively unhurt infant? What was she like? Happy, eager, demonstrative, open with feelings, quick to learn. If this behavior begins to change, this may well indicate stored hurt.

As we move from childhood through adolescence and into adulthood, we need to find ways to deal with hurts that may go way back in time and that can also recur throughout our lives.

We are all very familiar with the experience of getting physically hurt, from minor cuts and scrapes to broken bones and serious illnesses. We are all aware of the physical healing process by which our bodies, often with medical assistance, bring us back to a state of health. There have been, and continue to be, questions and speculation about the exact nature of this healing process, but there is no question that it does take place.

We have also all had the experience of being hurt emotionally. We experience loneliness, rejection, put-downs, loss of friends, death of those close to us, and many other forms of hurt. These emotional injuries can be as incapacitating as physical hurts, and they also require healing.

An old cliché says, "Time heals all wounds." There are indications that this isn't true. We know countless people who carry old bitterness to the grave. Everyday conversations are full of references to painful memories, unforgotten and unresolved. You surely have heard, "She was never the same after her husband died—she went downhill very quickly." Or again, "When his business failed, he seemed to lose interest in everything."

In fact, a dynamic set of processes is available to all of us, which we could label *emotional healing* or *unhurting*, that is very much more than simply putting lots of time between ourselves and the old hurt and trying to forget. It is perfectly possible and natural for us to recover completely from any upsetting experience. All of us have at least partially recovered from many such experiences, although this tends to become more difficult for us as we get older. The reason has nothing to do with "aging," but with social taboos on behavior.

What does the unhurting process look like? It is often easiest to see in children, as we have suggested earlier in this chapter. Janet, aged two, falls down the stairs. She is hurt and terrified. She runs to her mother crying. At first, she screams, perspiring, then sobs, and then, between sobs, she tells what happened. She continues to cry and talk for some time. She will point to parts of her body that hurt. If her mother touches them gently, she resumes crying. She might show her mother where the accident happened. If her mother has enough time and patience, Janet will relive the entire experience, feeling and getting rid of each painful feeling.

This is an example of what unhurting looks like. We know that this process has a beneficial effect because those who have a chance to feel the fear and hurt in this way in the presence of a loving and attentive friend function without the fear and hurt afterwards. The complete release will be followed by bright, loving, intelligent behavior. When Janet is done with her crying, she plays as contentedly as before she fell. If she doesn't have the chance to cry, she will remain upset and will try to set up situations in which she can cry. She may well carry a fear of the stairs for a long time.

We sometimes have difficulty listening to crying. We know that when people are crying they are hurting, and we believe that, if we can get their minds off of the subject and onto something else, we will stop them from hurting. This is well-meaning, but incorrect. It is *unhurting* that we are listening to, and we either allow it to happen, or the hurt gets stored and causes trouble later.

Josh, a two-and-a-half-year-old boy, came home from spending a weekend with his grandparents, whom he loves very much. He seemed excited about his weekend, but he also cried easily and frequently. That night he woke up crying and asking for his father. His father came to his bed, and Josh cried long and hard about a frightening experience that happened over the weekend. His grandparents had seen that he was upset and quickly distracted him. Now that he knew he was with his parents who would let him cry, the painful feelings resurfaced. After he cried for some time, he went on to talk of the fun he had had with his grandfather over the weekend.

The difficulty most adults experience in listening attentively to the process of unhurting is precisely the reason why we, when we become adults, have such difficulty unhurting ourselves. It has been thoroughly drummed into us that "Big boys don't cry," "You mustn't be such a sissy," and "That's enough now, dear. Here's a cookie." The message, whether it is nicely or harshly stated, is the same. The adults do not mean harm. It is just that the crying or the tantrum recalls all their memories of when they were stopped from crying. By giving the cookie, or threatening, or quickly suggesting another game, they shut off their own painful memories. The result is that, instead of releasing hurts quickly and easily as they occur and learning about the world in the process, we begin storing the hurts, which later impair our ability to function rationally, and we begin repetitive mistake-making. This is the key reason for all or most of the irrational behavior we see in ourselves and the people around us.

If we really do have an inherent self-healing process available to us which has been thus impaired, how can we be of help to each other in regaining the ability to heal ourselves? We all have memories of people who intended to be helpful to us but ended by failing completely. I have asked people to list things friends have done who were trying to be helpful to them when they were hurting. The list includes "giving advice," "taking care of me," "smoothing things over," saying, "Oh, I know. The same thing happened to me," or talking about their own, much bigger problem. Some, in despair, conclude that there really is nothing people can do to help each other, and that we must face our problems alone.

HELPING EACH OTHER IN HEALING HURTS

In spite of all these errors, it *is* possible for humans to be of real assistance to each other in healing emotional hurts. The self-healing process, to work well, requires the presence of at least one other human being who is capable of loving, aware attention. The child, as we have seen, works his own healing easily and spontaneously if given the chance. For most adults, it is more difficult, because, in addition to the hurt we are feeling at the moment, there is a long series of painful memories of being told to stop when we tried to heal ourselves.

To begin the healing process, we have to turn around the cultural taboo about displays of emotion. There are some cultures where it is acceptable for men to embrace and weep with happiness when reunited with old friends, and for women to be angry and show their anger. Most of us, however, have been heavily conditioned to keep our feelings a private matter. Therefore, we are never freed from the grip the feelings have on us. This is difficult for us and for the people close to us. A married woman with several children once said to me of her husband, "It's one of the biggest disappointments of my life that Bob has not been able to learn to cry." These old taboos tend to remain because they are reinforced by messages in the present. Later in the same conversation, the woman admitted that, "I think if my husband ever did break down and cry, I would feel like my world was coming apart." This information was clearly communicated to Bob even if it was never put into words, and had an inhibiting effect on his expression of feelings.

In spite of the pressure to live in secrecy with our emotions, feelings have a way of leaking out. Some cry over romantic novels, others at movies. Some yell at their favorite football team or unburden themselves to the bartender at their tavern. Men will sometimes take a friend out drinking and, after "having a few," will burst into tears and talk about how "my marriage is falling apart." Anyone who is a good listener is sure to be approached frequently by friends who have a problem they want "to talk out." In reality, they want more than this. They want a chance to unload the weight of feelings that makes their life feel so dreary. Because they are usually not fully aware of this, the conversation rarely extends beyond talk and perhaps a few tears or loud, angry declarations.

Anyone who wants to assist in the self-healing process must aggressively contradict this deep-seated assumption that feelings must be kept private. Assure the person who is hurting that it is the most natural thing in the world to want to talk about a problem and to feel all of the feelings connected with it.

To illustrate, let us visit Mrs. Rowell, who is deeply distressed by the break-up of her daughter's marriage. She finds herself in conversation one morning with Mrs. Slayton, a trusted friend. With much uneasiness and embarrassment, Mrs. Rowell brings up the subject of the separation. Let's assume that Mrs. Slayton is an excellent listener. She can tell that her friend is uncomfortable, but also that she very much wants to talk. Mrs. Slayton is not herself embarrassed by the subject. She cares deeply for her friend and has some confidence in her own ability to help. She is therefore quite relaxed, interested, and patient, but not over-eager. She gives her friend the space and time she needs to bring the painful subject up. In the meantime, she does *not* change the subject or steer the conversation in the direction of something "more pleasant." She simply waits, listening and smiling, looking warmly at her friend. Mrs. Rowell has reached the point of acknowledging that "it has happened," and, from that moment, has busied herself wiping the counter with a dishcloth and washing the top of the honey jar. Mrs. Slayton leans forward slightly and says gently, "Louise, this has really been weighing on your mind, hasn't it?" Mrs. Rowell puts the honey jar down, stares into the living room, presses her lips tightly together, and nods quickly. Mrs. Slayton says, softly, but without the least trace of distress in her voice, "Wouldn't it be good just to sit down and talk about it? I have plenty of time this morning, and I'd like nothing better." Still looking into the living room, Mrs. Rowell eases herself into a chair and looks down at the dish towel, rubbing it back and forth on the edge of the table. Mrs. Slayton smiles broadly and reaches across the table for her friend's hand. "Louise," she says. Mrs. Rowell glances in her direction and manages a quick, tight smile. "Louise," Mrs. Slayton continues, "we've been good friends for a long time. I think so much of you. And I know what a good mother you've been to your children." Mrs. Rowell shakes her head furiously and sobs begin. "No, no! That's just it. I haven't been. I'm not. How could I be a good mother when I feel the way I feel toward my own daughter?"

"How do you feel toward Judy?"

"I'm so angry! I'm so angry!" She throws the dish towel on the table and faces her friend for the first time in the conversation. She has said the thing that was hardest to say, and now the rest comes easily. She alternately talks and cries: she and Bert must have done something wrong, she has failed, she knew things were not right, etc. Mrs. Slayton listens. She doesn't critique or analyze or point out where her friend went wrong or try to convince her that really nothing is wrong at all. She allows her friend to feel every feeling, even the worst ones, without reproach or denial of the reality of the feelings. But she does not allow her friend to devalue herself. She allows her to feel the feeling that she has failed, but reminds her that she has always, without exception, done the very best she could. She allows her to feel the anger toward her daughter, because she knows intuitively that she must feel the anger and move through it before she can love her daughter again without qualification.

This is one example of how a friend can help a friend with the emotional self-healing process. What did Mrs. Slayton do right? She remained calm, caring, and interested. She did not try to hurry things. She was self-confident, and made it known that she expected the best possible thing to happen. She let her friend know that she cared about her. She was not distressed by her friend's problem. She empathized, but did not participate in the pain nor contribute her own feelings, which would have interfered with the process. She kept her friend on the track. She did not try to distract her. She watched for the hurt, and gently but persistently kept her friend's attention focused on it. She affirmed the goodness of her friend and insisted that she had done well in spite of her feelings to the contrary. She did not allow her to get mired down and lost in the hurt feelings. She reminded her, by reaching out and touching, smiling at her, that she was there and everything was all right in the present. Knowing that in the present she was safe and cared about made it possible for Louise to delve into the hurt feelings, feel them, and come out again.

What is the result of a conversation such as this? What good does it do? One such session will not obliterate the pain of such a difficult time, but it will make a start. In this fictional example, beginning to release the pain will make it more possible for Mrs. Rowell to talk with her daughter, to express her love for her, and to feel her love in return. It will make it possible for her to talk with her husband about the situation, and for them to evaluate together what is happening with their daughter and their relationship to her. It will help Mrs. Rowell to realize that she can reach out to friends for help rather than try to bear the whole burden alone. In general, she will feel less like a trapped victim of her feelings, and more like someone powerful enough to act intelligently and appropriately in the situation.

There is no need to stop with one session. Friends can do this for each other, even on a regular basis, with varying degrees of formality. The things that tend to stand in the way of such action are feelings which, when properly evaluated, have no merit, such as feelings of invading someone's privacy. There is such a thing as real need for privacy, but when you leave a friend alone who is hurting badly, you are, in effect, abandoning him, no matter what he says, since there is no way he can release the hurt by himself. There are feelings of embarrassment, feelings of inadequacy, feelings of hopelessness. None of these is a reason for not doing something. They are simply obstacles we need to overcome in doing what we see needs to be done.

An important final point should be made about helping other people with the healing process. If you wish to offer help in this way—and no doubt, despite your embarrassment and timid feelings, you do—you should be very clear about your role. You are a helper, an assistant. It is a *self*-healing process. You provide an essential ingredient—your attention, caring and interest. Without it, the person who is hurting would be helpless in the face of the hurt. But, with your presence, he is the one in charge of the process. He knows where he needs to go and what he needs to do. You have to watch carefully and make sure he does not wander off onto byways.

The healing of psychic hurt is genuine healing. We are not doomed, like old soldiers, to carry emotional scars to the grave. With the intelligent and caring assistance of friends, we can rid ourselves of the daily accumulation of hurts as well as the heavier weight of old distresses.

We have covered some of the essential points for the assistant in this process to remember. All that remains is to shuck off self-consciousness and give it a try!

12
Adulthood: A Growing Season

A common conception which people carry around with them is that we go through a formal educational process—high school or college for the majority—and, at about the same time in our lives, our physical growth slows up and stops, and, after this point, all learning and all growth stop! It may sound incredible, but this is how a great many people feel.

This is a *mis*conception for many reasons, but mainly for these three: the growth of emotional stability takes longer, the growth of wisdom takes longer, and the growth of the spirit takes longer than twenty or twenty-two years.

We are working against strong programming in our society. Here is some of it:

- Now you are sixty-five, and suddenly you need Geritol.
- Now you are sixty-five, and you are being retired from your job.
- Now you are fifty-five, and you will be retired in ten years, so you must already be slowing down.
- You are a grandparent, so you must be old.
- You have gray hair, so you must be old.
- There is a new generation of ideas and feelings, and yours are no longer valued.

That's pretty heavy stuff to overcome, isn't it? Well, we can, we will, and we must overcome it—our lives depend on it. People in middle age definitely can overcome this propaganda because they have begun to acquire some wisdom, they really have strong bodies, they have active inquiring minds, they have calm emotions, and they have a vibrant spirit *if* they choose to have these things. The sooner they make the choice, the better!

So, let us eat biogenically; exercise regularly and vigorously in all seasons of the year; read voraciously, learn eagerly, and watch TV minimally; put a little aside for travel; meet and talk to stimulating people; learn how other people live; meditate regularly, or use a regular relaxation technique; visualize ourselves as perpetually healthy, endlessly learning, and vigorously growing. Let's *be* what we visualize!

Then, let's have a look at the next three chapters for some other good ideas!

13

Positive Programs for the Human Mind

BETS ALBRIGHT

In an earlier chapter, we spoke about the vast amount of programming that is fed into our human computer starting even before birth. Since so much of this material has a negative effect, we need to find ways of removing the useless and destructive stuff and substituting positive, nourishing, valuable content.

If a computer can be programmed in one certain way, it can obviously be programmed in another, different way. We have spoken in some detail about the stages and types of programming that affect us as human beings, and about what programming does to the functioning human unit of body, mind and spirit.

There is one big difference between the human computer and its IBM counterpart: we *can* learn to reprogram *ourselves*. The more solid and rigid the input, the more difficult it may be to change its character. But it is important to believe firmly that it *can* be done—and unrealistic to say that it will be easy.

INFLUENCES BEFORE AND AFTER BIRTH

It seems unlikely that the fetus in the womb can resist the influences of negative programming. If the parents have unhealthy attitudes and habits during the gestation period, stress may well be coming through to the growing life.

But if the young mother, in cooperation with the father, thinks of herself and treats herself as a sound, beautiful, healthy vessel for the growing embryo, then surely the infant who comes into the world will have the best possible start. If love and caring are transmitted to the child from the parents during this time, then these seeds will grow as the infant begins its life in the world.

This is the ideal picture. Sometimes the child in utero cannot receive the concentration of positive energy from parents that is best for his growth. For example, adoptive parents need to give special love and energy to the infant who has been given up by his physical parents. I believe that this is quite possible to do, and I have seen exciting examples of young parents of an adopted child who begin programming the baby from the day they receive the news of his or her arrival. They know and understand the special needs, now and in the future, that their child will have.

I know a couple who began a book for their adopted son as soon as they knew he was to be theirs. They filled each page with the most glowing love, enthusiasm, and energy—and created a treasure and heritage which would be given to their special child just as soon as the right time came to tell him that he had grown in their hearts rather than from their bodies.

A good deal of emphasis has been given, in recent years, to the environment in which a baby is born. Harshness, bright lights, and abrupt actions do not start the infant on his world-journey in a physically or spiritually healthy state. New and gentler birth scenes will indeed begin the programming of an infant for well-being.

Parents of young children can do a great deal to help their child to think of himself—and to *be*, whole. As I pointed out in the chapter on programming the human computer, the world will deal more harshly with some children than others. But surely those who know from the beginning that they are loved and accepted just as they are and who are wisely prepared for the knocks that society will inflict later on will have a better chance of surviving intact.

Family life can, from the beginning, emphasize wellness, rather than illness. Parents can refrain from assuming or expressing the idea that crying necessarily means pain. It may just mean the need for extra cuddling or rubbing, or an infusion of strong thought-energy. If you continually think of your child as well, the child will more likely remain so. This does *not* mean that infants will never get sick; they do, indeed, need medical check-ups. However, it is certainly desirable to learn as many ways as possible to maintain a healthy environment for little children. This includes a study of proper nutrition, an attempt to keep mealtimes happy, serene, and pleasant, and an optimistic, hopeful, constructive, confident attitude toward the child's development. If the various stages of child development are studied and anticipated, less stress will communicate itself to the baby.

It is very important to use care in speaking *to* the baby and *about* the baby in its presence, even when you are convinced that she or he "doesn't understand a thing." The child will absorb a lot more than you think—so you have a wonderful opportunity to program this small but powerful computer wisely and positively.

As soon as your child is old enough to respond, begin to *listen* as well as speak. Now comes the real need to think about your child not just as a sometimes lovable, frequently trying little addition to your home but as a marvelously structured unit. There is the amazing physical body and its surrounding energy body, the mind with its left- and right-brain potentials, and the still quite untrammeled spirit. For some time, you have a very real responsibility for what you contribute to the programming. You will need to think about what is beginning to filter in from outside of the close family unit as well. There can be negativity bouncing off of visiting relatives and friends which you may need to divert and counteract as firmly as you can.

KEEPING A HEALTHY BALANCE DURING CHILDHOOD

If you keep in mind that your child is a balance of masculine and feminine, logical and intuitive, light and dark, gentle and strong, you will watch for influences that push the balance too far in one direction or the other. It is an exciting challenge if you think of it this way and forget that you can hardly *wait* for Johnny to hold his first baseball bat. If Johnny thinks of baseball as one of the fun things he can do with Dad or Mom, the results will probably be great. If he feels that Dad will love him less if he's no good at batting and prefers reading, the results will be clearly-stamped messages that he is inadequate.

As children grow a little older in a family where tasks are not assigned by sex nor given ratings as menial, boring, deadly, etc., but rather, challenging and *shared*, even if they aren't always a thrill—then the computer won't be cluttered with unnecessary resentments, dreads, and blocks against work.

The healthy-programming task becomes more complicated as the child spends more time outside of home—in school, or with friends and neighbors. It can be really helpful to talk with children about the influences that will enter the scene. Not all of the problems will be solved, but a shared awareness of what is negative and unhelpful, and an opportunity to talk over such things at home and to make decisions about coping with them will be very useful.

"Why do I have to color inside the lines and make things the color teacher says?" This question really requires action on two levels. At one point, parents need to become involved with the teaching methods used in the schools. At another point, they need to help their daughters and sons to deal with frustrations that will cause negative programming. "You could show the teacher that you know *how* to color neatly—and then ask for some paper so that you can do the picture the way you would *like* it to look" is one way to answer.

Dealing with the influences of the media is not easy. Parents should certainly be aware of what their children are reading in magazines and hearing and seeing on radio and television. It can be fun to talk about these things. Evaluate them together. Parents can explain what is behind the advertising, and can also listen carefully to what the children think and feel about what they are taking in.

If children are treated as healthy, vigorous beings—given simple, wholesome foods and plenty of exercise and rest—they develop positive habits of thinking about themselves. If there are relatives in poor health, discussion can take place of why the health breakdowns have occurred, with emphasis upon the fact that this is not something that will automatically happen to them because it happened to Aunt Mary. Instead of issuing continual warnings about the dangers of catching cold, the positive-programming parents will emphasize all of the things that are done in the family to keep colds to an absolute minimum. If colds begin, there are routine, natural ways of keeping them short-lived. If the parents have faith in these, so will the children.

USING CREATIVE IMAGINATION

I believe strongly in teaching children as many ways as possible to use their creative imagination. Parents can teach simple meditation techniques which help children to relax, to go within, and to visualize. Techniques are being used by doctors and psychotherapists to help stressed children cope with illness and emotional problems. These have been very successful, and I feel that it is advantageous to teach such techniques to well children also. Learning to relax and to visualize is a wonderful and helpful habit, and is very simple for children. It is useful in everyday life and it can be put to instant use if special stress situations occur.

Books are available which help to teach meditative skills and which deal with visualization techniques. Some of these are listed in the bibliography at the end of this book. The skills are not difficult to teach or to learn.

With young children, learning can be made into a quiet game. Sit down with them and do some simple exercises to relax and get comfortable. Let them make suggestions for this! Then close your eyes, ask them to do the same, and begin to take a visual trip. Remember that if it is to be relaxing, it mustn't be too exciting, just pleasant and peaceful.

Many ways exist to visualize the body as relaxing. You can allow "warm, golden light to flow through a window in the top of your head. Let it bathe all of your body from the head down, soothing, healing, softening." You can treat each part of your body as a bag full of sand and empty the bags, letting the sand flow out slowly. You, or your children, can think of many more ways! Once relaxed, you can take a trip to a sunlit field or to a forest glen.

When the child becomes used to this technique, he can begin to find his own way. He can be encouraged to meet and talk with imaginary people during his inner-seeing sessions. Perhaps he will have conversations with animals or people, and, in the process, solve some problems that have been worrying him.

For simple meditation that does not involve any problem-solving but simply relaxes and centers and opens the way to new levels of consciousness, a child or an adult can use a word or short phrase which is repeated. She or he can think of one flower nodding gently or one number repeated mentally.

Inward-going, inward-being, and inward-looking are all healthy and health-improving. If a child is going through frequent periods of illness, encourage extra meditation times. Work at a visual technique to deal with the health problem. If a youngster thinks in terms of bad guys and good guys, then it is no trick to visualize the good guys wiping out the sickness, which is pictured as the bad guys!

This visual imagery technique has been used by Dr. Carl Simonton of Fort Worth, Texas, in working with children suffering from cancer, but it can help in much less severe cases. If a child has a broken leg, urge the young patient to picture the two ends of bone being put very neatly together and then growing *quickly* into strength and wholeness. There is really no end to the ways in which these positive energies can be marshalled to help physical problems and mental attitudes!

If children are helped in these ways, they will surely grow up less victimized by programming and much better equipped to deal with what does slip into the computer when they are unaware!

I have emphasized particularly in this chapter the importance of positive programming before birth and during childhood because so many negative programs originate during this period. Obviously, many people will reach adolescence and adulthood with a heavy load of useless or downright destructive programs which must be dealt with in order for them to achieve wholeness. The adult who has an unhealthy, negative self-image needs love, help, and support before the unity of body, mind, and spirit can become his personal reality. Many of the chapters in this book deal with ways in which the accumulated blocks in the healthy flow of life energy can be dissolved.

All of the techniques I have described as positive programs for the minds of children will work for adults. As I have said, the longer negative programs remain in the computer, the more work it will be to replace them with healthy, positive substitutes. The basic essential for success is the belief that change *is* possible, and that a technique is not the whole. It is only a part of the process of learning to activate the healing, change-making ability that is within us all.

14

Exercise and Yoga: Regaining Our Place of Power

DEVAKI BERKSON

Many recent articles and books have been fantasizing, analyzing, and eulogizing all the myriad aspects of yoga and exercise. The world of exercise and yoga, which was once framed in a caste-system matrix where the big guys played football and the thin hippies sat cross-legged, is elbowing for room for diverse and daring participants. It is just as possible to witness thin-legged women prancing joyfully and deer-like through marathons as it is to see hefty businessmen conquer a head-to-knee yoga posture. Boundaries are not being bound to, but are being bumped and stretched and expanded to whatever the fortitude and mysticism of the participant can energize. We are in the midst of a mass exodus, a return to a sincere enjoyment of living in one's own body. Most people are uncomfortable inside themselves, and some of us want out—out of feeling this way, that is.

Now this is a very profound statement with far-reaching implications. And it is a perturbing reality that many people exist from moment to moment, year to year, in the permanent home of their body and mind and don't feel good about it. How many people do you know who aren't embarrassed by certain physical or psychological weak links in their beings which they consequently hide by clothing and/or behavioral mechanisms? Why is it that so many of us are uncomfortable inside ourselves?

110

WE HAVE GIVEN UP OUR CONTROL

One powerful answer resounds: We have given up our control.

To whom and why? The answer is twofold. Firstly, we have given up the lifestyle that puts one in control. We live lives of less and less motion, sitting for longer and longer periods with less time spent outdoors. Though life is movement, we wonder why we are dying. Secondly, we have given up our control by handing over our power and decision-making to higher commercial institutions whose priorities are money, not people. Their profits wage control over our appetites, our consumer habits, our life-style habits, and our self-images. Mega-industry and psychological marketplace warfare have successfully convinced most women that they are forever undesirable unless they look stick-thin all the way from here to there, and smell synthetic, "kool-aid" sweet all the way from up north to down south. We are cajoled to be skinny and foxy; and, at the same time, we are lured, encouraged, and bombarded to eat this, eat that, watch television, and snack some more. It's "Catch 22" all the way. The marketplace now becomes an avenue in which to optimize profits rather than optimize humanity. We are caught in a spiritually limited and downward spiral of reflexive behavior. We must snack a Big Mac because, each time we see the Golden Arches, a Pavlovian jingle rings in our ears and we are wooed and won by the neon sirens. Too few educational processes along the way emphasize personal body and mind control, self-awareness, decision-making, and wisdom. Life becomes a collection of manipulations by elite institutions; and, when we buy dingle bars and fiz-wizz colas to spend hours sitting in front of the never-ending TV shows, we are unaware that we have given up, as Carlos Castanedas phrases it, our "places of power" and of courage.

George Sheehan, noted marathonist and cardiologist, once said: "You can live your entire life in the United States and never know you're a coward." These words are very intense because they echo so truthfully. They intimate that many of us are satisfied to give up our "power" and live in a gray zone of convenience. But this is precisely what the new exercise-yoga-mind revolution is all about: leaving the gray zone and exploring new edges, getting back our personal power, our personal joy, and our harmony. There are many edges in our lives today, stress-filled "edges," where we bump boundaries and then retreat. However, there are very few ways in today's world that we can expand these edges through personal perseverance, and revel in the fruits of our success. Exercise and yoga offer one way.

OUR INTUITIVE HERITAGE

It is truly interesting that we are having to *relearn* all the things that were *intuitively* known by our ancestors. Movements which were integral parts of their tasks kept our ancestors in motion and challenged. In our society, we have no more use for these movements, such as water-carrying, house-building, and ritualistic dances. In making our lives convenient, we have lost some of our daily life-dances; we are left stiff and confused. It's the same in all things: In agriculture, we have to learn methods of growing through books and institutions, while our ancestors knew these things instinctively. Part of the sacrifice for our cement-condominium-consciousness has been to give up some of our intuitiveness. What the new exploration and use of exercise and yoga is about is retrieving our intuitiveness, regaining our (as the psychosynthesis people call it) seat of wisdom. This is a place within us where we truly know something because we know it without having learned it. It puts exercise in a shamanistic order: movement is life and brings one in touch with more life. George Sheehan says, "Never trust an idea you come upon sitting down." No matter how successful you are as president of a corporation, if you're always sitting, what you are controlling is the corporation, not *your* life.

"GOOD" STRESS

In trying to regain our power, our intuition, and our confidence in our bodies, we ask ourselves how we can do this framed in a society where stress abounds. People are becoming aware of stress and examining ways to ride its razor's edge. It's sharp and it's slippery, but it can be useful. There are two types of stress. One is destructive, and one is constructive. Harmful stress is stress which is translated to tension. This inappropriate tension is debilitating. Most of us, when we hear the word *stress*, think of divorce, anger, traffic, bureaucracy, didactic institutions. Then there is the second type, called creative stress. This is stress which can be usefully transmitted to work for us, not against us. Today, various methods of movement, diet, and mental mechanisms that, in themselves, require stress-filled and demanding practices constructively reward us by putting us more in touch with our places of power: growth, awareness, challenge met and conquered, and enjoyment and pride in mind and body.

Stress is always in our lives. Why not use it creatively and successfully? Movement, through yoga and exercise, is a creative stress which inspires a powerful rhythm in which to dance to our place of power once again.

BENEFITS OF EXERCISE: THE PHYSICAL

We all know exercise makes us feel good, but few of us know the fascinating details. Here are some facts with far-reaching implications you can ponder.

Whenever *exercise* is mentioned, it is understood to stand for *aerobic* exercise. This means exercising the heart with an adequate oxygen supply. Cardiac output during aerobic exercise produces significant beneficial changes in the entire cardiovascular system, and heart damage is unlikely. *Anaerobic* exercise, in this chapter, signifies inefficient oxygenation. This is running when you wish you weren't, with heavy legs, loss of breath, and build-up of lactic acid in the muscles (stiff muscles due to extra hydrogen combining with pyruvate and making lactic acid). Anaerobic energy production takes over when aerobic reactions are insufficient to meet the energy demands of the exercise. As the level of lactic acid builds up in the blood and the end of aerobic resynthesis is seen, heavy-duty fatigue is reached. (Some athletes' abilities during competitions may be due to their high tolerance for increased lactic acid levels.[1]) The aerobic condition is associated more with health, while anaerobic is associated with disease. It is vital both to maximize one's "aerobicness" and to keep limber and sensitive by doing stretching routines such as yoga. Aerobicness builds up the cardiovascular system, while yoga refines, protects, and expands the whole body. Limber, toned-up muscles protect joints and are less susceptible to injury. Tight muscles can pull bones into slightly inefficient positioning, make the body more susceptible to ligament and tendon damage, and decrease the vascular and neuronal supply of the whole body, on all three levels, physical, mental, and spiritual. Thus, a well-balanced program gives respect to both aerobic exercise and yogic stretching.

Exercise Retards Aging

Dr. H. Shock defines bodily deterioration in terms of the loss of physical working capacity due to the heart's reduced ability to deliver sufficient blood and oxygen to the working muscles and tissues.[2] Many factors contribute to this reduction. One of them is an increase in catabolic hormones, which influence larger elements (like proteins) to break down into smaller ones (like amino acids). Coffee, sugar, and other artificial stimulants encourage catabolic reactions within the body. Increased catabolic activity can increase cholesterol resynthesis in the body, as well as other stresses on the body.[3] Salzman found that the heart's duties are challenged negatively by catecholamines, compounds that stimulate a sympathetic response like epinephrine and novepinephrine.[4] They found that physical exercise can help prevent excessive catabolic stimulation.

Many studies reveal how aerobic training restores cardiovascular fitness in the elderly, defying time and our social concepts about older people. A University of Toronto study found that exercise improved the level of fitness of an old person to that of a person ten to twenty years younger.[5]

After studies sponsored by the Administration on Aging (AOA) and conducted under the auspices of the Andrus Gerontology Center in Los Angeles, Herbert deVries, Ph.D., concluded that "physical conditioning through a careful, well-planned exercise program can be expected to improve the health of the cardiovascular system through several routes. Most importantly, it improves the heart muscle itself." He goes on to enumerate the following benefits: reduced blood pressure, reduced tension (which, in turn, normalizes blood pressure), decreased body fat (reducing coronary-disease proneness), and improvement of the ability to breathe (this important point shall be discussed in just a while).

The implications of these findings are far-reaching. They show that God is merciful. A little effort brings a lot of reward, and a little exercise brings a lot of youth.

I am reminded of a nightmare once experienced by the articulate biochemist Dr. Jeffrey Bland. He dreamt of the person who gets into his car in the morning and never gets out of it. He drives to McDonald's for breakfast on a bun and has the meal served in through the window. He starts the car and proceeds to the drive-in bank, the drive-in dairy stand, and then stops for a snack at Taco Bell, where another plastic tidbit is pried through the window. Off again, this person drives from one square edifice to another, never having to leave the car or use his legs. He grows larger and larger. A Burger King here and a Dairy Queen there—he continues to grow until, like a liquid, he begins to assume the shape of his car, fat, pouring like mayonnaise, through the steering wheel, over the back seat, onto the floor. He becomes the shape of the car. He is his just dessert.

Yet, even this victim, with exercise and effort, could rapidly shed the results of his "sins"; with exercise and yoga, he could find himself shrinking back to increased health, longevity, and cardiovascular functioning. The famous Thaddeus Kostrubala, M.D., who runs marathons and holds marathon clinics, began as an overweight skeptic who had to drink vodka to gain the courage to reluctantly don his running shorts. Now he's a happier, thinner, running maniac.

God is compassionate, and exercise is one of the pleas to which nature is most responsive and respectful.

Exercise Clears Cholesterol from Our Arteries

HDL (high density lipoproteins) are to our vascular system what our garbage collectors are to our garbage. Every Thursday morning, they start out from the liver and drive to the most intimate lining of our arteries, pick up some cholesterol and carry it back to the dump where it can be recycled (hydrolyzed and degraded) into bile acids. HDL's are good guys.[6] New uses of the clinical laboratory for prevention reveal that the higher our levels of HDL's, the less our chances to develop coronary heart disease. Exercise increases HDL's. HDL levels are found to be higher in extremely physically active people such as runners, hikers, etc.[7]

Most people still naively fear cholesterol as the big "bugaboo" in arteriosclerosis. This is not the total picture. Our bodies make almost 70 percent of our cholesterol. We make so much cholesterol that, unless we had an appropriate avenue to clear or degrade it, in just a short while we would end up as 170-pound walking cholesterol sandwiches. HDL's play a necessary part in the clearance of cholesterol and its conversion to bile acids.

Thus, exercise helps maintain the integrity of our arteries and keeps coronary heart disease further away than arm's length abeyance.

"Putting Out" Energy for Exercise "Begets" You More Energy

We all remember how our energy is produced in those parts of our cells known as the mitochondria. It is here in the mitochondria that our energy is stored in the form of ATP (adenosine triphosphate). It is as if we had our money in the First National Bank of Oregon and each mitochondrion were a different branch. Our currency is ATP, and, when we need some energy to get something done, like make a dandy hormone or stack some amino acids together to make a few more curls in our hair, we go to the bank and draw on our reserves. We draw out this ATP and it gives up a phosphate group. Spending a phosphate group produces energy. Thus, ATP contains a vital unit of energy.

Exercise increases the body's ability to regenerate ATP. When one starts to condition the body, there is an increase in the array of glycolytic and Krebs-cycle enzymes. This means more mitochondria, which means more energy. Exercise can increase glycolytic enzymes by a function of three.

This is an incredible statement of health. The more we exercise, the more mitochondrial action we produce, the more energy we actually have. This means more energy to repair, heal, and clean out garbage.

Disease can be redefined as a process of anaerobicity, and health as optimal aerobicity. Sustained physical effort, especially at 70 to 85 percent of maximum capacity, has the most beneficial aerobic and mitochondrial effect. Health can be seen as having the energy system of billions of cellular doctors capable of optimal repair and service. The more you move, the more life you beget. The real Zen is finding the stillness within movement, not only sitting still.

Exercise Protects Against Coronary Heart Disease

Mechanisms by which physical activity may reduce the occurrence or severity of coronary heart disease are shown in the following list:[8]

EXERCISE INCREASES:	EXERCISE DECREASES:
coronary collateral vascularization	serum lipid levels, triglycerides, cholesterol
vessel size	glucose intolerance
myocardial efficiency	obesity, adiposity
efficiency of peripheral blood distribution and return	platelet stickiness
electron transport capacity	arterial blood pressure
fibrinolytic capability	heart rate
red-blood-cell mass and blood volume	vulnerability to dysrhythmias
thyroid function	neurohormonal overreaction
growth hormone production	strain associated with psychic stress
tolerance to stress	
prudent living habits	
joi de vivre	

This is an impressive list of the fruits of exercise. I especially like the "joi de vivre." The more you move, the more you groove; no doubt about it.

Exercise Affects the Breath, the Cerebral Spinal Fluid, and Hormones

When we breathe, our sacral and cranial bones move. They move in specific directions on inhalation and exhalation. This statement of physiology is at the interface of professional disagreement. However, citations in the literature provide validation. Cranial motion has been studied by Upledger.[9] Retzlaff related cranial movement to the activity of the heart and respiration.[10] Yogis have presented the information for thousands of years that the breath has revitalizing effects on many systems of the body. Yoga teaches that, as one breathes, there is movement up and down the spine which affects our glands and our states of consciousness. Medical ego may be currently unraveling and arguing about the beneficial aspects of breathing; yoga, faith, and common sense have known of these things for thousands of years. (Isn't it usually the case!)

As we inhale, the sacral base moves backwards and the cranial bones elongate and rotate.[11] Of course, this movement is in millimeters. Connected to these bones is the dura mater, the hard connective tissue covering the brain and spinal cord. This layer of tissue attaches to the sacrum at its axis of movement, and it also attaches to five places on the skull. As we breathe, this dura mater is rotated, and our bones move. There is controversy over whether the dura is moving the bones, or the bones the dura. But this movement affects the production of cerebral spinal fluid (CSF). This marvelous fluid surrounds the central nervous system and has been shown to carry important hormones and to communicate with other systems.[12] Fryman states that "CSF moves the cranium; respiration and movement move the CSF."[13] Cerebral spinal fluid feeds and protects the brain and spinal cord and is referred to by the yogis as the sacred fluid. This holy nectar is thought to affect our major master glands and, thus, to exert far-reaching effects over many bodily processes. Thus, movement and respiration "pump" and cause more production of CSF, giving another dimension to exercise, yoga, and the breath.

BENEFITS OF EXERCISE: THE SPIRITUAL

Yoga as a Therapeutic Tool

Much has been written these days about the emotional and spiritual highs of exercise[14] (an excellent example is Valerie Andrews' book, *The Psychic Power of Running*). People are discovering how successes in exercise extrapolate into one's life. However, not many of us are aware of the therapeutic aspects of yoga postures beyond limbering, relaxing, and thinning. Mr. B. K. S. Iyengar originally developed his method of yoga for the Indian army to "tone and toughen" the soldiers. However, he has redefined yoga by marrying its disciplined, almost ballet-gymnastic type attributes, to its medical and psychologically therapeutic qualities. He uses yoga as an arena to activate the glandular system as well as conquer psychological barriers. He is well known in India for working with muscularly disabled and semiretarded individuals, and, through yoga, enabling them to partially regain bodily control and self-image. Various postures, or positions, are used to excite and develop various bodily and psychological functionings. For example, the inverse postures incite assertiveness and courage. Most of us are afraid of disorientation, or being upside-down. When students need to work on conquering fear, they are given upside-down poses, such as head and handstands. Backbends require strength and pushing against the floor to lift oneself up. Assertive poses are usually easier for men. Assertive qualities are reinforced in men in our society. The forward-bending poses, such as head to knee, or the opening poses, such as legs spread wide with head to the floor, require fluidity and receptiveness, less aggression and more bending. These are usually difficult for men. Men working on these attributes are assigned specific programs of these poses.[15]

Felicite Hall, an excellent teacher at the San Andreas Yoga Center in Palo Alto, views various muscular systems in the body as correlated to various mental defense mechanisms[16]. For example, tight hamstrings express the emotion of having had to do many things one didn't really want to do, such as sitting at a desk for long hours. Psychological anger is seen stored in the calves (couldn't kick when wanted to), and emotional closure and lack of confidence are expressed as tension in the inner thigh or adductor muscles. The list goes on and on, and yoga postures to open these muscle groups are seen as affecting these mental attributes.

Yoga as an Edge Extender
We all have edges—edges of how far we can bend forward, edges of how far we'll take risks, edges of our dietary philosophies and boundaries. Joel Kramer, a unique and probing California Yoga teacher, teaches yoga as an edge extender. Our edges can be places of powerful confrontations depending on how we face them, and how we choose to explore and stretch them. Edges can be as powerful as any university education. Kramer teaches, for example, that our edge, in a head-to-knee pose, is that point when we are bent over to our maximum position without strain. He then advises us to "hang out" here for awhile, to take a look at this place, to notice if you are goal-oriented and your type A personality is begging for you to strain further toward your knees and toes. He inspires the students to be here, right now, and then, when the edge is fully explored, to extend it with the use of the breath: Breathe in and out, and, on a slow exhalation, let the breath move the body further; by doing so, the breath, without effort, extends the edge.

The emphasis is on effortlessness, allowing the breath to initiate movement and expansion. His comments ring true in yoga as they do for all exercise and life dances:

As soon as we drop the ambition and get into exploring our tightness, the conflict between what we are and what we want to be dissolves, and that brings a physiological relaxation . . . to be accomplishment oriented in yoga is to remove the energy from the process. . . . For me, the doing of yoga is learning how really to tune into the feedbacks, to the energy. . . . Yoga is adult play; and, like child's play, it involves a great amount of energy, but no effort. . . . The effort of goal-striving actually works against us, because it tightens us. . . . What I am saying is that when one becomes alert to the nature of ambition, one sees its destructive qualities and its binding nature. When one sees this, clearly, ambition becomes less interesting. Yoga can teach you about this in a very intimate way, both physically and psychologically.[17]

It's almost impossible to read these words and not feel humbled by the potential of yoga and exercise and to be honest as to our own ways of utilizing them.

BEING OUTDOORS IS MORE THAN FRESH AIR

Exercise can get one outdoors, into that wonderful space many of us watch wistfully through glass squares. Most of us are aware of the beneficial effects of fresh air, but not many of us realize the influence of natural lighting *striking* the eyes.

Our pineal gland acts as a photo-sensitive electric eye and is stimulated by light upon the eyes. Recently, citations in the specific literature are coming out, drawing correlations between health and pineal gland activity. For example, *The Lancet*, Oct. 14, 1978, p. 814, presents "the hypothesis that diminished function of the pineal gland may promote the development of breast cancer in human beings."[18] Dr. John N. Ott, in his *Health and Light*, discusses many beneficial effects of lighting on health and many adverse effects of unnatural or decreased lighting, such as arthritic problems and hyperactivity.[19] The well-known Dr. Bernard Jensen, at his Hidden Valley Health Center in Escondido, California, recommended that all his patients "sun" their eyes daily for the beneficial effects on the glands. This effect occurs in outdoor natural light even if the sun is covered by clouds.[20]

Thus, as you move and breathe outdoors, you are exponentially escalating your vitality, health, and well-being.

I had always thought of myself as born stiff and as more of a head person than a body person. The past nine years of yoga and now exercise, especially running, has expanded my self-image and world-life view. I know that I am who I am because of how I live, breathe, move, and co-create with God. I am dynamically always changing, being reborn, and bumping my edges, less with egg on my face, but more with joy in my heart. My edge, my foreground of today, is my background of tomorrow. Anything and every-thing is possible.

15

Making Friends with My Spirit

JOHN E. NUTTING

When I think of my spirit, I see myself living in an old New England farmhouse with the finished-off living rooms and kitchen at one end and a procession of sheds, ells, and drafty additions that have been built on the other end over the past 150 years. I live easily in the finished-off section of the old place, busy with the tasks of survival, accomplishment, and compassion.

There is constant activity in my end of the house. People come and go through the mud room into the kitchen. Messages arrive over the phone; the mail and the newspapers assault me daily, and I do my best to answer. I am plugged into a vast network that has uninterrupted access to my attention and energy.

My responses arise from deep convictions about the human family, and much of my initiative is devoted to the development of groups of folk who want to organize their efforts on behalf of their sisters and brothers.

My life in my end of the house is mostly spent in being available to others, reacting for others, and making sure that I have honored the requests for service or succor that come to my door.

Such a life is attractive and rewarding. It becomes frantic and terrible when the askings far outpace my ability to do much that is effective in response. There are, however, very few gaps in this life; usually it's complete and satisfying.

I'm sure I could live out my days moving about in only the finished-off section of my house. But such has not been the case.

Snowstorms have kept people from the door. Power outages and ice on the lines have stopped the ringing of the phone. Some days, letters and newspapers have not arrived, and I have been denied their delicious and demanding agenda.

My children have grown. Their askings have diminished, and their voices have lowered considerably. My wife and lover of the past two decades leaves the house for work, for bowling, making her own responses to the glittering world of involvement, achievement, service, and self-development.

So there is quiet. There is time to hear the clock tick. There is solitude, and even my dog sleeps in the middle of the day.

This means I am occasionally relieved of the need to respond, and I do not always need to consider the dynamic of some group. There are hours lately when no one uses my minutes and no budget is being projected. Obligations have been met—either well or poorly, but they have been met. Even my boss says, "No more work out of you. Go home. You've done enough."

This makes me ready and ripe for exploration and discovery. I find myself moving about the house. At first, I become more familiar with the rooms I live in every day. Then, after a while, I wander out through the ancient door that leads to the sheds at the other end. I remember my childhood Saturdays when I would rummage about that part of the house. It's been many years, however, since then.

THE FORGOTTEN TENANT

As I poke about those unused, unfinished, and nearly forgotten rooms in the far end of my house, I am surprised to find that a tenant has been living there all these years. If anyone had asked, I would have said, "That part of my house is vacant. We don't live there. No one does, except a few mice, an occasional bat, and some other creatures we don't want to know about."

But my spirit lives there. He's the forgotten tenant.

He's been living quite comfortably behind that unopened door, making no demands, calling for no attention, carrying on an existence I have neither known nor noticed. But there he is, a resident in the unfinished end of my house.

Having rediscovered my spirit, I find that he's rather shy. He's quiet, thoughtful, and gives the impression that he will wear well. I also get the feeling that he will have some surprises for me should I visit him again.

That's the way its been since I first opened the door and began to spend a few hours with him. During an early visit, we agreed that my body was too large. My stomach hung over my belt so that it covered up my Vermont Morgan Horse buckle. We decided I should lose weight, largely in the interest of vanity, somewhat in the interest of better health.

We took on this task together. After several years, nearly twenty pounds are gone. Our method has been to go hungry. When my stomach hurts for food, I know I'm on the right track. During times of hunger and denial, my spirit has called me a liar as I tried to cheat the scale. He has sworn at me when I've eaten three popovers slopped with butter. In the long run, however, my spirit has convinced me that less food can become my way of life. Now I can wear turtleneck sweaters with pride because my belly no longer hangs out disgustingly distended.

Now and then, a day comes when I have cleared my desk, made all my phone calls, and marked it "D-O" (day off) in my date book. In winter, my spirit gets very restless. He wants us to move around, get some exercise, go outdoors.

Because of his prodding, I prepare for cross country skiing in the vast woods behind my house. Onto my skis and into the forest by myself: that's the way my spirit moves me. Together we explore the untracked, ungroomed, unknown, and mysterious stands of hardwood and spruce that come almost to my back door. Challenge and dappled beauty meet me at every new glide of my waxless skinny-skis.

As my spirit and I move about the forest, I recall scenes from my boyhood, thirty years ago, in northern Minnesota. In that other time and place, the same spirit and I went through woods on skis, awed by the same wonders of atmosphere, terrain, and snow. Time and distance blend as my spirit and I pick up where we left off over threescore years ago. He befriends me with these ancient and satisfying continuities.

MY SPIRIT COMES A-VISITING

Once I have opened that door and befriended my spirit, he grows a bit more aggressive. Occasionally, he knocks on the door from his side and even wanders over the threshold to visit me. He keeps bringing up ideas, visions, possibilities, and new creations for me.

Lately he's invaded my mind with a whole new way of looking at the history of America. He's given me, the Anglo-Saxon intruder, the uncomfortable label of exploiter, land grabber, and defiler of the native Americans.

There are times when I wish my spirit would retreat to the dusty sheds of the unfinished part of my house. I have come to see, however, that my spirit and I are friends now. Before, I was more his keeper and warden. Now, he is no longer an unknown, silent tenant. I could not evict him even if I wanted to. He is a permanent resident who makes suggestions, demands, and an occasional joke.

I am eager for future adventures with my spirit. Having become reacquainted with him and discovered weight loss and woodland touring, I am impatient to discover what lies ahead for both of us.

News of tragedies may come through the mail, disasters may assault me over the phone, and conflicts may shatter the peace at my end of the house. Terrible events may break into my comfortable and finished-off living space. These dark times are expected, even though unwelcome.

In the time ahead, I look forward to moving closer to my spirit. He will be needed to keep me from becoming closed to novel, creative, risky, and demanding ways of doing things. He will be needed as a companion through the dark nights that will drop on me as I live with zest, passion, and a lust for accomplishment.

I think I'll soon take the door to the back shed off its hinges. With so much traffic between me and my spirit, it will just be in the way.

I am going to take the phone off the hook every now and then. I'll unplug the television and ignore the mail. Then my spirit and I will take our boots off and warm our feet at the fire. Perhaps we'll even doze a bit, complete in the sense that it's good to be, and very good to be together.

16

Attuning to Our Nourishment

BETS ALBRIGHT

ay this food, prepared with love, be shared and enjoyed in love—and may it contribute to the perfect unity of body, mind and spirit."
Hands meet around the table for a moment before the meal begins. All at the table are aware of the energy in the simple, wholesome food, as well as the strong life force in the atmosphere of love and sharing. There is much more likely to be joy and laughter at this meal than bickering and complaints, and the participants will leave the table feeling satisfied and refreshed, rather than heavy and ready for a nap!

There was a *Saturday Evening Post* cover by Norman Rockwell some years ago. It showed, as I remember it, an elderly woman and a young boy, with heads bowed and hands folded, saying grace in a small restaurant. Onlookers watched with puzzled tolerance. For many, blessing the food is only a childhood memory—or a strange rite observed by a few; but actually it makes wonderful sense!

The thing that impressed me most on our first visit to the Findhorn community in Scotland, was the act of attunement. This involves holding hands for a moment and centering thoughts on the activity ahead. We attuned before meetings, before work projects, before driving a load of rubbish to the local dump in a battered pickup truck, and before eating.

But why? What's the point?

It would be so simple if we could write out a neat prescription for the perfect diet and promise that, if it were followed, good health would be restored and maintained. It would help if all

126

foods bore neat labels; "eat me," or "don't eat me." We know that food is important—we have been told often that "You are what you eat," or "Food is your Best Medicine." Fine. But it is so easy to become bewildered by the vast amount of material that is spoken and written on the subject of nutrition. The authorities contradict one another in a most authoritative manner, and, as the books pile up around us, we wonder where the real truth lies.

As confusion mounts, we are driven to begin a sifting and sorting process. Are there threads that run through all of this information and tie some parts of it together? Can we build something that will enable us to live long, healthy lives, enjoying our food and helping others to do the same? We believe that the answer is Yes! What, then, are the materials with which to build good eating habits? Do we need to study biochemistry to survive?

We know it is possible that a plant may be fed and watered, placed in the sunlight—and it still may not thrive. We know people who partake carefully of foods in the prescribed food groups each day and who are still totally lacking in vibrant health.

We have seen bits of plant life that push through incredible obstacles and live, despite the lack of supposed essentials. There are people who apparently eat the wrong foods and appear to do well. The implication is that life is sustained by something more than the obvious.

In his chapter on healing, Paul Solomon speaks of the X-factor, the love and caring essential to the activation of the healing process. It is not difficult, then, to accept that there is an X-factor in nutrition as well, something other than the chemical content of the food and the biochemical activity that takes place when the food is eaten.

ENERGY AND NOURISHMENT

Each of us has an energy body surrounding our physical body. This is not a new idea. Diviners (dowsers) and sensitive people have known it for centuries, and many scientists have now come to accept that this is so and are trying to identify this type of energy. More recent studies indicate that the foods we eat have energy in varying degrees just as humans do. Kirlian photographs*

* A Russian named Kirlian developed a process using a special generator and photo paper—but no camera—to "photograph" energy fields. These pictures show astonishing energy patterns emanating from food, plants, humans, etc.

of loaves of whole grain bread show glowing energy patterns. Similar pictures of white bread with additives show almost no radiation of energy.

According to Edmond Bordeaux Szekely,[1] who has written extensively about the ancient Essene communities, basing his writings upon long and painstaking research of material from the Dead Sea Scrolls, foods can be divided into categories on an energy basis. There are first, biogenic (in Greek, life-generating) foods, such as seeds, whole grains, nuts, and legumes which can be germinated to mobilize their dormant life forces and thus create and generate new life.

Next, there are bioactive foods which can sustain the human life forces well even though they are not able to generate new, living organisms as the biogenic seeds can do. These foods include uncooked fresh fruits and vegetables.

The third category consists of foods which are neither life-generating nor life-sustaining, but which slow down the life processes in the organism. This would include cooked foods and foods which were not fresh. This category Szekely calls biostatic.

For the fourth category, which includes food containing harmful substances, such as chemicals, additives and preservatives, and foods which have been refined and processed, Szekely uses the word biocidic, life destroying.

Whether or not one adopts entirely the Essene way of eating, this is a fascinating approach to thinking about our foods and worth using when we make our choices.

FOOD AND LOVE

I believe strongly, although I cannot prove it in a laboratory, that when we prepare food with love, and serve and eat it in a pleasant atmosphere with people who have joined in blessing the food, or attuning, we have helped to activate the energies in our food so that what we eat will be used by our bodies to maintain the balance that is good health. I also believe that if we feel, as is sometimes inevitable, that the food before us is lacking in life energy, we can hold our hands over it and ask that we be channels for supplying the lacking energy. Obviously, it would not be wise to use this method carelessly in order to expect poor food to do the trick for us on a regular basis! We need to work continually to restore the balance. We need to use ourselves as tuners or dowsers or diviners, however you wish to say it, to tune into the information available to us about nourishment.

To fellow-seekers after good nutrition we would say, Do not be lured by diets that claim to be the sole solution. Eat simple foods in moderation. Eat as much food that is grown in your area as you possibly can. Find a balance between cooked and raw food that suits you and your family. If you try eating less meat, you may soon find that you need and want only small amounts.

Dr. Land's chapters on the art of nourishment are full of help and wisdom, and at the end of this book you will find a list of good books which may be helpful to you. Eat well! And remember that you are feeding your body, mind and spirit!

17

Food and People: Two Systems Interacting

DONALD LAND

Most simply described, a system is a collection of "things" that interact in a certain way. The "things" may be parts of the body, parts of an automobile, parts of a city, the animals, insects, and plants, etc. in a forest, or other smaller systems. The interactions may be described mathematically, chemically, mechanically, politically, spiritually, and so on. A less simplistic notion comes from realizing that complex systems can *not* be reduced to a sum of the parts plus a sum of the interactions; the things, or components, described alone or out of context, do not have the same meaning as components described in terms of the interactions in which they engage. The more complex the system, the less likely that we can describe any component out of the context of its relationships with other components.[1]

THE SYSTEMS APPROACH

Two major goals emerge in analyzing any system:

1. To describe the system as accurately as possible. The more we know of the components and their interactions, the better we understand the system.
2. To use the system in a predictive mode; i.e., to study the effects on the *total* system of altering one or more components or altering the ways in which the components interact.

This can be done by manipulating an actual system (for example, removing an organ from an animal or adding certain insects to an

130

ecological system) or by manipulating a *model* of the system which is described mathematically or otherwise.

One can find ecological, urban, world, interplanetary, or intercellular systems described in the literature. Current interest in holism is an extension of systems thinking, although it has not *formally* grown out of systems analysis. This interest does, however, represent an attempt to view the human being in its totality, affecting and being affected by all that it comes in contact with. The human being can be seen as a complex system of body, mind, and spirit which we attempt to understand through many disciplines. It is, also, a small *sub*system in a much larger system. We are connected in complex ways to each of the others in our species, to other species, to our creations, our activities, our music, our dance, and our environment. If the adage "We are what we eat" evokes crude thoughts of being made of cheese, beans, and rice (or their component parts), the speculation that "We are what we do" or "We are what we think" evokes images of a much more complex system of body, mind and spirit interaction.

SYSTEMS THINKING AND PERSONAL RESPONSIBILITY

As we begin to *think* more in terms of systems, our abilities to be aware of the consequences of our existence are enhanced. We are put in closer touch with events that we mutually influence, and, thereby, are put more in touch with our sense of responsibility. Personal responsibility has become a major theme in our current attempts to understand how best to promote health.[2, 3]

The systems approach to nourishment requires that we broaden our concept of nutrition from the traditional concerns with isolated nutrients to the larger concerns with the wholeness of food, as well as with all the factors in the maintenance or destruction of that wholeness. We will next look at food itself from a systems point of view, followed by considering the body as a system, and finally, the interaction of the two systems.

THE TRADITIONAL VIEW OF FOOD

If you inspect a food label, or a table of the nutrient values in food, you generally will find values for up to five minerals (Ca, P, Fe, Na, K) and five vitamins (A, C, B_1, B_2, B_3). These generally are referred to as the key or major nutrients. Most courses and texts in nutrition put emphasis on these nutrients and their deficiency symptoms. The idea of a key nutrient is born out of the drug model in which a single substance is seen to be "active" for a single purpose. Vitamin C is a key nutrient because of the classic cases of scurvy that show obvious symptoms of extreme deficiency of Vitamin C (or at least of citrus); likewise, beri-beri and pellagra show symptoms of deficiency of Vitamins B_1 and B_3 respectively.

Nutrition Teamwork

Roger Williams is most articulate in emphasizing that teamwork is essential in nutrition. He is, in effect, making an appeal for a *systems* approach to thinking about vitamins and minerals: "Because this [teamwork] principle is neglected, a wholly unscientific concept has been widely accepted with respect to what a nutrient may be expected to do."[4] In other words, vitamins, like medicines, are tested for specific action on specific diseases. The problem is compounded when this linear thinking is reversed: if a single nutrient is not effective against a specific disease, it is deemed worthless, or, if specific clinical symptoms are not noticed with low levels of a nutrient, then "the need in human nutrition is not established."

Ross Hall further clarifies the situation: ". . . unless a system can be defined in which a single disease problem is identified with a single chemical, the nutritional scientist does not have a workable experimental system."[5] Vitamin C (ascorbic acid) is thus seen as a suitable replacement for citrus (the whole fruit) because it is active against the *symptoms* of scurvy. Reductionist, nonsystems thinking leads us to equate Vitamin C with citrus without regard for the context of its source or of its use.

Williams makes several notable points:

- while no nutrient by itself is an effective remedy for any common disease, the nutrients acting as a *team* are probably effective in the prevention of a host of diseases
- there is no evidence to suggest that nutrients *not* commonly listed in tables are not key nutrients
- food composition tables give only fragmentary information which is easily misleading, especially when processed and fortified foods are involved

• "nutrition surveys" reflect the same neglect of the teamwork principle.[6]

What becomes clear is that, in order to begin to get a complete picture of the nature of the functioning of food, we must learn to see food as more than a list of identifiable nutrients.

Optimum Nourishment

Another serious deficiency in nutrition education and the public understanding of the function of nutrients is in the concept of *optimization*. Discussion of nutrients generally centers around the Recommended Daily Allowances (RDA) which are based on the amount of a nutrient necessary to prevent clinical deficiency symptoms. A more useful approach to understanding nutrients and the total value of food might be to focus on the amounts (as well as the context) that produce *optimum* functioning of the human system. The concept of optimizing becomes at once a systems question, including the idea of nutritional teamwork as well as that of a *health*-oriented approach to nutrient utilization.

Looking beyond our current inventory of essential nutrients, it is difficult to imagine that, before the end of the century, we will not have discovered or recognized a substantial number of new nutrients. These probably will fall into one of two groups:

1. Newly discovered compounds
2. Known compounds whose nutritional importance will be discovered

Also, these compounds may be nutrients themselves, or may be potentiating factors. However, the difference may be virtually nonexistent from a systems or teamwork point of view. As we develop our systems sense of food, it becomes apparent that there exist many factors that contribute to the wholeness of food, i.e. to its ultimate value in nourishing the human body. Ballentine[7] presents an enlightening insight from the perspective of Ayurvedic (traditional East Indian medicine) nutrition.

The Limits of Chemical Analysis

One begins to get the picture that perhaps our human senses, if working properly, may be the best tool for analysis of food after all. In spite of the many benefits, most analytical methods have severe limitations, in that—

1. ingredients or components may be detected, but processes or interactions among components remain obscure and can at best be inferred;
2. the methods of analysis, with rare exception, require that the component be observed out of its natural or original context.

The inference of function from structure may be misleading, as is pointed out by Ross Hall: ". . . nutritional science has mistakenly assumed that the function of a vitamin is encapsulated in its chemical structure."[8]

Technology Is Not Science Is Not Technology

It is common public misunderstanding that science and technology are essentially equivalent. They are related, but not equivalent. In simple terms, technology is concerned with making things work, whereas science attempts to understand *why* they work as well as to be able to *predict* events within a given system. Although science may lead to a particular technology (for example, the science of polymer chemistry preceded the plastics industry), very often the technology develops first and may or may not be based on an underlying science; for example, the technology which developed the battery eventually led to the science of electrochemistry. Many technologies have developed through the ages that were not based on scientific understanding, such as extraction of metals from ores, fermentation of alcohol, and production of ceramic utensils, to mention a few.

The public assumes that the processing and manufacturing of food is based, to a large extent, if not in its entirety, on food science in which all underlying principles are thoroughly understood and tested. On the contrary, much of our production of food is the result of a technology with little or no underlying science of nourishment. As a result, we understand little about the effects on human health of fractionating our food, of mechanically, chemically, or genetically altering our food, of chemical additives and pesticides, or of totally synthetic food. The gap between nutrition science and nutrition technology will narrow only as public scrutiny leads to demands for less technology and more understanding of the implications of rearranging our food supply.

BODY, MIND AND SPIRIT: A COMPLEX SYSTEM

A major theme in the holistic health movement is the integration of body, mind and spirit.[9] Each functions with the other as a whole system that is not reducible to the sum of its parts. A major goal in our new awareness is to begin to understand the nature of these interrelationships.

In the cells of the body is where nourishment begins. Even (or *especially*) at this level, we can learn the lessons of providing optimum nourishment. Roger Williams reminds us of two irrefutable facts at this level: (1) a properly nourished cell will function optimally; (2) a cell improperly nourished will malfunction or eventually die.[10]

Our respect for one lowly cell will probably be enhanced when we realize that it is a microcosm of the entire world (sometimes I wonder if not the whole universe) with "complex chemical transformations, . . . designing and making blueprints . . . assembly lines . . . transportation systems . . . sorting, pumping, and streaming . . . feedbacks . . . communications systems . . . sewage and disposal systems . . . pollution control mechanisms."[11] Collections of cells become organs, and interfunctioning organs become systems of organs—respiratory, digestive, reproductive, endocrine, blood, lymph, etc.

In the Oriental view of the body's interfunctioning, these systems nourish and control each other according to ancient laws.[12]

As we recover from years of having separated the body from the mind, new treatises appear on the ability of our thinking to influence reality.[13] Norman Cousins reminds us that "enough verifiable data have appeared about the ability of the human mind to play a major role in overcoming illness to make this entire field enormously attractive to laymen."[14]

Mental functioning includes all of our senses of perception: sight, hearing, taste, smell, touch. We are learning much about the influence of our diet and lifestyle on these senses.

There are many notions about what constitutes the spirit.

Bloomfield describes the spirit as "that which sustains harmony among all parts."[15] The concept of spirit may also include consciousness, environmental sensitivity, and a sense of connectedness to all parts of the universe. Many thinkers have equated total consciousness or enlightenment with total integration, harmony, or balance of body, mind and spirit.

More evidence of body, mind and spirit interaction comes from studying a range of phenomena from "spontaneous" remission of illness and placebo effects to sorcery and psychic phenomena. As we learn more about mental and emotional symptoms which are related to nourishment patterns, we, on the other hand, also learn that lack of love, touch, and general stimulus can produce physical illness.

In considering nourishment of the whole person, it is important to realize that so-called psychological aspects can be both a cause and an effect of dietary patterns. Restlessness, nervousness, anxiety, and irritability, as well as changes in the senses of taste and smell, can be symptoms of an imbalanced diet, but also can lead to behavior patterns which produce dietary imbalance. It is often impossible to separate cause from effect.

Eastern systems of medicine (Oriental, Ayurvedic) recognize, as an integral part of their design, the relationship between functions of specific organs and specific aspects of a person's emotions and mentality. In Ayurvedic medicine,[16] the duodenum, or solar plexus, where carbohydrate is broken down to release the sun's energy, is related to the fiery aspects of a person's physiology, emotions, and mentality. The liver seems to be related to depression and to the mind, the adrenals to chronic tension and anxiety, and the thyroid to nervousness and exhaustion. The pancreas and stomach are related to angry feelings, the colon is associated with nervousness, fearfulness, and anxiety, and emotions can over- or under-activate the digestive system. According to the Oriental Five-Element theory, excess anger injures the liver, excess joy injures the heart, excess worry injures the stomach, excess grief injures the lungs, and excess fear injures the kidneys.[17] This system also shows how certain emotions counteract each other, and which emotions tend to stimulate or depress various organs and their associated emotions. Further, it has been suggested that the glands are the interface between the body and the mind.

COUPLING WITH OUR SUPPORT SYSTEM

As we consider the complex relations that characterize the body system, a clear picture begins to emerge: that physical, mental, emotional, and spiritual nourishment are required and that there is substantial interplay among these requirements. A supportive system of nourishment must be able to promote total well-being by providing optimum nutrients, both known and unknown, while minimizing the inclusion of toxic materials.

Laszlo developed the concept of a system as an irreducible group, irreducible in the sense that we would agree that *reduction* to its parts (taken separately) and the interrelations among parts (also taken separately) is hopelessly complex.[18] The reductionist or "scientific" approach can only—at least for the moment—promise us an incomplete, perhaps misleading, view of the group (system).

Only from a total body-foods system picture can we begin to make sense of what we observe in terms of food patterns and corresponding illness patterns. We can begin to develop more comprehensive cause-effect relationships for problems such as heart disease that focus on broader concerns than, say, the amount of fat or cholesterol we eat. Disease is seen more clearly in terms of a weakened organism, and is not limited to outside influences. The idea of teamwork in nutrient utilization is no longer seen as a special case of cooperation but as a natural result of a systems viewpoint. This new systems picture should provide guidelines to help us design more workable experimental systems. At least we would better understand the limitations of biochemical experiments which study the functions of natural components—vitamins, minerals, carbohydrates, etc.—taken out of their natural environment. If we really want to study the effects of nutrients, drugs, poisons, microbes, stress, or fasting on human beings, we should have some idea of the difference between healthy individuals and unhealthy ones—in the total sense—before we select our experimental population. And we should, perhaps, not present our results except in this light.

In so doing, we will no longer be able to define adequate nourishment in terms of lists of nutrients and fractionated foods. Our dietitians, nutritionists, food manufacturers, physicians, and food-service managers will have to reevaluate the nonsystems which develop foods for the market place and menus for hospitals, nursing homes, schools, correctional institutions, and other facilities which we intuitively *know* do not produce health.

Recognizing Whole Food

The link between the body and food systems is expressed most directly through the senses. All of them are involved: taste, smell, sight, feel, and sound. However, another of nature's ironies prevails: our senses and organs must also be nourished. We are now in the midst of perhaps one of the first adult generations who for the most part have never seen food grow, but, worse, have been conditioned to recognize and prefer only manufactured, artificial, or modified tastes and flavors. We are reminded that "body wisdom is probably not fostered by the consumption of deficient foods."[19] Ross Hall comments on our ability to select wholesome food saying, "When food technologists began to separate nutrition from palatability, they also undermined the ability of the senses to assess the quality of the food—man's senses no longer guide him in his choice of food items."[20]

One of the effects of coupling with an artificially produced food system is that the senses are no longer a part of the body-food system in a way that allows us to be attracted to wholesome foods. Instead, our senses tend to lead us toward those foods to which we are most addicted or otherwise attracted.

The missing and added ingredients in our food can affect not only our sensory experience with the food, but can directly affect our perception and evaluation of it. When our mental and emotional functioning is out of balance, so are our food preferences. It seems that the imbalanced craving for certain foods, as well as the rejection of others, tends to push us further down the spiral toward increasingly unhealthy habits. So, what we eat affects what we eat. Not surprising!

However, the situation is not, and should not be, hopeless. We as consumers are reeducating ourselves as to the value of foods. In the first stages, we are learning—not necessarily through our senses, but by substituting intellectual awareness—specifically which foods have been depleted of fiber, vitamins, and minerals; which foods contain potentially harmful additives and pesticides;

which animals have been subjected to which drugs and which toxins; which foods have been fractionated, restructured, synthesized, picked before ripe, or cosmetically dressed up. From changes brought about by this awareness, our senses begin to return to us.

In the second stages, we may notice an increasing appreciation of the source of our food. Many of us reflect on this in a spiritual or meditative way. We also may begin to develop renewed senses of proper handling and preparation of food. We will eat more slowly and more reflectively. Sharing a meal may, on occasion, even become a spiritual sharing. Finally, we begin to regain our sense of how we feel as a result of what we eat: peaceful, attuned, heavy, energized, too full, etc. The complex interplay of body, mind, emotions, and spirit begins to turn into an *upward* spiral: instead of being sick getting sicker, we are well getting "weller."

Diet and Disorder

There is not much dispute these days that most "physical" ailments are diet-related. Even conservative opinion recognizes that six out of ten major causes of death in the United States are diet-related. The notion that mental and emotional functioning is related to diet (as well as to many other aspects of our environment and lifestyle) is relatively unexplored, but is currently commanding a great amount of attention. Difficulties with perception, judgment, and functioning seem to come from a spectrum of factors which includes heredity, prenatal malnutrition or toxicity, traumatic deliveries, early postnatal malnutrition, and subsequent environmental influences ranging from diet and stress to lack of exercise and relaxation.

The critical point here is that, contrary to our usual practice of helplessly relinquishing our bodies, minds, and responsibility to the medical technicians, many of these factors can become matters of conscious decision and control.

The following are four ways in which mental and emotional illness can occur from diet patterns that result from having lost touch with our natural support systems:

1. *Deficiencies in B vitamins*[21]

    Deficiencies in several of the B vitamins can produce emotional or mental symptoms. Most Americans do not eat foods high in the natural B complex, such as organ meats or whole grains; on the other hand, we consume large amounts of processed carbohydrates which demand certain B vitamins from the body's stores for their metabolism. In addition, we are subjected to varying amounts of stress, which puts additional demands on B-vitamin stores. Using the RDA's and the add-up-the-nutrients model, dieticians, nutritionists and physicians lead us to believe that we are generally well supplied with B vitamins. The prevalence of the following kinds of symptoms leads me to question seriously whether we have *optimum* intake (even considering the fact that none of these symptoms is exclusive of other causes):

B_1 *(Thiamin)*—Loss of appetite, depression, irritability, confusion, loss of memory, inability to concentrate, fear of impending doom, sensitivity to noise.

B_3 *(Niacin)*—Anxiety, depression, fatigue, apprehension, illusions, visual and auditory hallucinations, hyper-acute sense of smell, dulled sense of taste (perceptual changes similar to those produced by schizophrenia)

B_{12}—Symptoms ranging from poor concentration to stuporous depression, severe agitation, and hallucinations.

Pantothenic acid—Volunteers fed a diet deficient in pantothenic acid became easily upset, irritable, quarrelsome, sullen, depressed, tense, dizzy, and numb.

2. *Vitamin dependencies*[22]

In contrast to vitamin deficiencies, which are acquired, vitamin dependencies seem for the most part to be genetically transmitted. Evidence has been presented to suggest needs by certain individuals for some vitamins and minerals of up to 100 times the average need. An individual whose needs are high, but who has an average diet, may show the same symptoms as an individual getting less than an average amount of vitamin. A supportive concept known as biochemical individuality has been developed by Roger Williams,[23] which suggests that many individuals vary widely from the average or "normal" requirements.

Large amounts of vitamins and minerals have been used with varying degrees of success in the treatment of schizophrenia, childhood schizophrenia and autism, learning disabilities, mental retardation, alcoholism, drug addiction, neurosis, allergies, and hypoglycemia. These therapies are often most effec-

FOOD AND PEOPLE: TWO SYSTEMS INTERACTING **141**

tive when used in combination with conventional therapies.
3. *Cerebral allergies*[24, 25, 26]

Symptoms of mental and emotional disturbance can be produced by allergic-type reactions to food that center in the brain. A wide variety of foods and food chemicals have been investigated for their tendency to provoke these reactions. Very closely tied to allergic reactions are food addictions; many foods or food chemicals seem to be both stimulants and toxins at the same time.

One of the more common theories related to the notion of "ecologic mental illness" is Feingold's linking of hyperactive behavior to certain artificial flavors and colors, as well as to some naturally occurring salicylates.[27, 28]

4. *Hypoglycemia*

Hypoglycemia has become a topic of extreme current interest to health and medical practitioners. Commonly taken to be synonymous with low blood sugar, it might more properly be equated with *unstable* blood sugar: it can be defined as the inability of the body to regulate its own sugar levels. Its etiology, nature, and dietary treatment have been discussed extensively.[29, 30, 31, 32, 33] Of interest here is the fact that a long list of mental and emotional symptoms commonly occur, are frequently misdiagnosed, and are often thought to be due to psychiatric disturbance. Systematic dietary treatment is often quite effective in alleviating symptoms (that is, restoring balance). These range from anxiety, nervousness, and irritability to forgetfulness, violent temper, and suicidal tendencies. One theory of the causation of these problems focuses on insufficient glucose supply to brain cells.

SIMPLE CAUSE-AND-EFFECT THINKING

The commonly accepted medical concept of a "disease" depends on being able to establish an etiology (cause-effect relationship). If causes and symptoms can be established, the disease can be described based on these. Generally, symptoms can be put into the following two categories:

1. General symptoms which may result from many causes—for example, headaches, fever, lassitude, anxiety

2. Specific symptoms that tend to be direct clues to identifying the disease

The apparent success of the allopathic medical model[34] is based on the treatment of infectious disease, or sicknesses which result from the ingestion of *obvious* poisons. Diagnosis was most successful when enough specific symptoms were present to give adequate clues. Simple cause-effect relationships could be established. This situation not only expedited diagnosis and treatment, but gave the patient a simple idea of the cause of the illness and encouraged the patient's submission of his body, mind, and responsibility to the physician.

In the United States today, we are faced primarily not with infectious diseases or obvious poisons, but with a vast spectrum of degenerative disease and not-so-obvious poisons. Symptoms tend to be mostly type 1 (above), the causes many, the clues short, and the degeneration highly interactive. For example, a weak digestive system may show a multiplicity of symptoms occurring over a long period of time, may have many causes rooted in our dietary habits and mental states, and may cause eventual difficulties in *any* system in the body. In short, an increasing number of causes and symptoms make cause-effect relationships, and, therefore, diagnosis, very difficult to establish. The real culprits often go undetected. The very concept of "diagnosing an illness" becomes less and less useful or effective in promoting health.

The situation seems to be epitomized by conditions such as hypoglycemia. Medical opinions range from the assertion that it does not exist—based, it seems to me, on a reluctance to give up the 19th century simple cause-effect model—to reports of some 200 physical, mental, and emotional symptoms correlated with it, nearly *all* of which can be produced in many other ways, i.e., have many "causes." It has been suggested that this increased misdiagnosis of illness itself causes illness.[35] The stigma of being told you have "disease" often creates a mental picture that, in fact, renders the patient not only helpless, but sicker.

Examples of simple cause-effect thinking are often manifest in the treatment of patients. Cholesterol consumption is often seen to be the sole or primary "cause" of high blood-cholesterol levels. Patients have been put on low-cholesterol diets with no consideration of the total body balance or of dietary factors which may *de-*

crease these levels. Patients with kidney stones may be put on diets which eliminate or minimize calcium intake, again with no consideration of the source of imbalance which produces the stones or of the fact that calcium is an essential nutrient. These are examples of thinking patterns and attitudes which lead to the mechanistic practices and habits promoted by our traditional medical view of disease, a view that constitutes a serious violation of the systems view of the process.

Treating Symptoms and "Causes"

Western medicine has been substantially criticized for its almost total disease-orientation and its treatment of *symptoms* by use of drugs and surgery. This, in part, has led to an increased focus on treating the "causes." However, even this new focus often falls short because of its emphasis on *simple* relationships and its failure to associate cause with total, holistic body balance. Muramoto gives us the Oriental perspective: "Traditional Oriental medicine does not conceive of the body in parts; it considers the organ a part of the whole, and disease a deterioration of the entire body system."[36] The essential value of understanding the causes of disease in a holistic context is that we are encouraged to prevent and eliminate disease by the proper selection of diet and life-style. When we understand that it is within our power to make ourselves well, we often *do* it. A true systems approach necessarily is based on the oath of Hippocrates: "The treatment shall do no harm," or, by implication, the least harmful treatment should be given the highest priority.

It frequently has been pointed out that the symptoms of disease are the body's early warning signs of imbalance. The signs may indicate acute short-term imbalances or chronic imbalances. Airola, for example, stresses: ". . . disease, as we know it, is a self-defensive effort of the body to restore impaired health."[37] He sees most diseases as having the same basic underlying categories of causes, all related to our lifestyle: faulty nutritional patterns, constant overeating, excess protein, nutritional deficiencies, sluggish metabolism and consequent retention of toxic wastes, environmental poisons, toxic drugs, alcohol, tobacco, emotional and physical stresses, and lack of exercise, rest, and relaxation. This approach to categorizing illness puts the emphasis directly on a *weakened* body rather than on assault by bacteria or poisons.

Just as our view of illness has tended to be mechanistic, our view of food and the body's vital processes that assimilate it have tended to be expressed in terms of lists of ingredients and isolated processes operating in separate systems. The notions of vitality and life in the body cannot be described or understood solely in terms of its chemical reactions, nor can vitality and life in food be reduced to a list of nutrients. To imagine that the functioning of a nutrient in the body can be understood solely in terms of its molecular or atomic structure is to ignore not only the conditions under which the nutrient is presented to the body, but also to ignore the conditions of assimilation. We tend to think of nutrients as drugs—molecules that bombard a certain "section" of the body and cause it to "do" something. Even here, our fascination with simple cause-effect relationships has led us to perform literally millions of scientific experiments to determine, for example, the effectiveness or lack of effectiveness, of a particular nutrient for a particular purpose. We try, for example, to determine whether vitamin A "cures" acne, whether vitamin C "cures" the common cold, and whether vitamin E increases sexual performance. But in few, if any, experiments of this sort does there seem to be a careful attempt to determine the health or balance of the experimental group.

"What Does Zinc Do?"

This question is typical of our tendency to think mechanistically of vitamins or minerals as drugs. The function of nutrients in various subsystems of the body and the resultant interactions of those subsystems with each other can be understood only in a holistic or systems sense. We may note that zinc relieves acne or promotes healing, or is important for growth, or intensifies a sense of taste or smell. But the real importance of zinc begins to be apparent only when we realize that zinc is present in *at least* ninety different enzymes, and is important in cell division as well as protein synthesis. Only in this complete context does the importance of nutrient deficiency become real.

Armed with this perspective on the importance of *whole* foods, we can get to the practicalities (and problems) of our own personal nourishment from both a defensive and positive point of view, and of nutrition as a therapeutic tool.

18

The Practice of Holistic Nutrition

DONALD LAND

n "Food and People" we looked at the standard American diet (SAD), which, to some extent, has been exported to non-American countries as well, including the Orient. We also saw the evidence that the human body is a system of complex systems, and that simple cause-and-effect thinking is inappropriate when dealing with the effects of one complex biological system (food) on another (the human body).

Armed with those basic pieces of information, and with a few others we have discussed, we can consider the practice of *holistic nutrition*. This deals with how we as individuals can provide ourselves and those we love and prepare food for with optimum nutrition toward the goal of vibrant health.

First, we will look at what I call the art of defensive nourishment, which is the art of avoiding foods and chemicals relatively low in the production of usable energy and/or relatively high in toxicity. Then, we will proceed to what I think of as positive nourishment, or the art of adding foods to our diet which produce high energy and radiant health.

Finally, we will consider nutrition as a therapeutic tool. This is a complicated subject which I would like to try to make a little simpler for all of us. Here again, we run into the basic concepts of health, "disease," balance, and healing which need to be re-sorted in the context of nutrition.

A lot of conflicting information exists in the field of nutrition, but a few basic principles will help us evaluate what we read.

From that point on, much of our decision-making will be individual, based on our sensing of our body's needs.

DEFENSIVE NOURISHMENT

The art of defensive nourishment is the art of skillfully avoiding foods and chemicals that have the potential of weakening the body or impairing its functioning. It is truly an art in the sense that it involves developing insights into the body's functioning, creativity in diet, and sensitivity to the results. An integration of many concepts, it is a totally personal matter and involves skillfully placing oneself into a complex picture of nourishment in much the same way that an artist integrates a particular color, image, or texture into his total work.

Personal Choices

Defensive nourishment means exercising personal choices. It can begin when we are able to free ourselves from the restrictions of parents, teachers, institutions, ghettos, and old ideas. Individuals can be categorized according to those aspects of life over which we have control. For the first five or ten years of our lives, most of us eat what we are given to eat. School lunches and other institutional food may physically limit our choices. Poverty, limited access to alternatives, lack of awareness, the influence of advertising, cultural patterns, and peer pressures constitute additional restrictions to choice. If the majority of our energy is devoted to bare survival, looking for the next meal, or just getting something that will fill the stomach, defensive nourishment is hardly a reality. We often are unmotivated because we see no point in changing diet; then we lose sight of our role as co-creators of our own health.

Practicing the art of defensive nourishment means willingness or ability to *go out of our way* to shop, develop new eating patterns, find information, go to meetings, challenge assumptions, and acquire the assertiveness to deal with intimidation by defenders of the status quo.

Personal Power

But it's not all give. There's plenty of take. And we're back into that circle again: We have to make certain choices to guarantee our personal power, but we need to exercise that power to motivate us to make the proper choices.

As in going through most changes, I think it is important to begin with small successes. We are too easily overwhelmed, frustrated, and willing to give up on our power: "It's too much—I may as well eat what I like and enjoy it." But if we *at least* do those things which *can* be done through diet, I think it's a step toward regaining our power. Certainly to *some extent*, dietary changes can provide us with the freedom to function better, to think more clearly, and to make better decisions. Every choice of food we make is a statement about how we choose to use our power. Total health involves many factors, as the theme of this book states. But, for many of us, diet will be the easiest and most direct entry point.

Defensive Tactics

Let's try to get to some specifics. Each individual must establish his own defensive tactics or goals: for most individuals, it's easier to tackle one or two goals at a time. Listed below are some steps to take that roughly match my own priorities. I have listed them in the order in which I think it is easiest to develop awareness, from the gross and obvious to the subtler concerns.

1. Avoid excess sugar, salt, and fat.
   Sugar, in my opinion, is the number one health problem in the United States. It has been strongly implicated in tooth decay, diabetes, obesity, heart disease, and hypoglycemia. Salt is almost as ubiquitous as sugar, and fat accounts for 45 percent of the average American caloric intake. Testimonies against sugar have become legion.
2. Avoid potentially harmful chemicals.[1, 2, 3]
   It is very difficult to know which particular chemical will damage the body at any given time, but the first line of defense is to be aware of—
   possible carcinogens;
   other additives suspected of being dangerous;
   artificial flavors and colors—especially in the case of hyperactive children;
   pesticides in produce;
   drugs and chemicals in meat and dairy products.
3. Avoid fractionated, synthetic, and restructured foods.[4]
   This list includes processed grains: white flour, white rice, and many commercial cereals.
4. Avoid excess meat and dairy intake.

The problems here range from excess protein intake and toxicity due to undigested animal products to toxic drugs and allergic reactions.
5. Be aware of poor food combinations.
For example, don't eat raw fruits with raw vegetables. Poor combinations can lead to a multiplicity of digestive disturbances. Often, the ill effects of food can be minimized by simplifying the combinations that we eat.
6. Be aware of highly acid foods.
It is recommended that the major portion of our food intake consist of alkaline foods.

It might be a good idea to set your own priorities. Begin slowly. Devote an entire period of time to working on one area, then the next, and so on.

Beyond this list, the best defense is a good offense.

POSITIVE NOURISHMENT

Positive nourishment involves adding health-building foods to our diet. For most of us, it involves some kind of transition to more carefully thought-out foods, recipes, ways of eating, or ideas about food. For some of us, it means simplifying our diets; for others, it means more complexity and more possibilities. But always, it means creativity. It may mean more work for some, less for others. But always, it will give us the feeling of doing something *positive* for ourselves and those we feed. Some of us proceed cautiously, others full steam ahead. But what keeps us *all* going, at whatever pace, is the attitude that it *can* be done, *should* be done, and will make a difference in our lives.

Positive Attitudes

That's the key: the attitude. Take a look at the list below. How many times have you expressed or heard any of the negative attitudes that I often hear? Under each negative attitude, I will list some corresponding positive attitudes that could be developed. The difference between those who begin to take responsibility and those who don't is expressed in the two sets of attitudes.

· We don't *really* eat much sugar.

Maybe we eat more than I think; let's start investigating.
I wonder what would happen if we tried to eat even less.

- Our diet is not so bad.
  We can still improve; let's see where.
  Maybe by other standards our diet is not that good.

- I'll never be able to give up————
  Well, maybe I can cut down.
  Maybe I'd feel better if I did.
  Maybe, if I find other things that are exciting, I'll change my habits.

- It costs too much to eat well.
  Maybe we *can* work out a healthy diet on our budget; other people do.
  It will cost more, in the long run, *not* to eat well.

- *Brown* spaghetti—yuccch!
  OK, I'll try it.
  Maybe mixed half and half with the white stuff will be OK.

- Who has time to cook everything from scratch?
  OK, I know the time I put in will be repaid in many ways.
  I'll find the time.
  It doesn't *have* to take a lot of time.

- My kids will *never* eat raw vegetables.
  Maybe they'll eat vegetables if they're fun and attractive.
  Maybe I can get them involved.

By some quirk of socialization or manipulation, 80 percent of my audiences, professional or otherwise, are women. And they are mostly the ones who do the buying and cooking. A common observation on my part involves women who go home to try new ideas but run head-on into mates with conservative, insecure, and closed attitudes. Macho attitudes. Got to have meat on the table every day, the redder the better—red meat equates with manhood. Green vegetables, salads, etc. are rabbit food. (That they are also gorilla food may or may not score you any points in your arguments.)

I've seen families take a range of approaches, from sneaking in whatever wholesome food won't be noticed,[5] to involving the whole family in discussing, understanding, planning, and enjoying the diet transition. Somewhere in between may lie the approach that suits your situation.

Positive Family Activity

Here are some of my ideas on things to do to get your family involved.

· Help to raise the general consciousness of your family with information and ideas.
· Begin with each family member's health problems and research how diet can help.
· Look for anecdotes and examples of positive results, especially with people you know.
· Share cookbooks, recipes, and ideas—especially books with *attractive* pictures.
· Consider seducing them with party foods or desserts that incorporate nutritious ingredients.
· Give each person some responsibility in the whole scheme.
· A Saturday afternoon cooking party might become an institution in your family.
· Experiment with *new* foods or old foods prepared in *new* ways.

Eight Important Points in Managing the Transition

Several years of experience working with students in cooking skills courses have brought up the following eight points of emphasis:

1. *Go slowly.* Don't think you have to make all the changes right now. What matters is not how much you accomplish, but that you are at least moving forward.
2. *Integrate new ideas into your life-style.* As long as you continue to think of food and ideas about food as something apart from your total life, you will probably not make much progress. Changing your diet means, in essence, changing your life-style, even if only slightly.
3. *Avoid the unfamiliar at first.* In the beginning, stick with familiar foods; soyburgers, seed milk, and strange-looking casseroles

usually don't appeal to virgin palates.

4. *Learn to accept and live with confusion.* If, in the first months or years of your transition you find yourself quite confused, you are quite normal and well on your way. I make a point of this because confusion is inevitable; but don't let it discourage you. *Stay with it.*

5. *Study.* For some good reading, select from the list in the back of this book.

6. *Find some support.* It's tough to go it alone. Seek out friends or groups who are also involved in changes. Or start a support group of your own. You can share ideas, recipes, frustrations, and successes.

7. *Go to a supermarket and study it.* Go there when you are *not* shopping. Study labels and prices per pound. Develop a sense of what you can buy in the supermarket that is acceptable according to your *current* standards. Shopping will then be less confusing and you will buy less junk (which, of course, is the first step toward getting food companies to replace it with wholesome food).

8. *Go to a natural food store and study it in the same way.*

Back to the Kitchen

Okay, enough talk. I hope that, by now, some part of you is wound up enough to head back to the kitchen with more enthusiasm than you had the last time you were there. There is a wide range of things you can look forward to doing. Each of you is on, or will take, a different path, but you will probably find yourself involved in at least one of the following:

Preparing more meals from scratch;
Modifying old recipes with more wholesome ingredients;
Learning new techniques, such as stir-frying, sprouting, blending, and drying;
Using nontraditional foods, such as tofu and miso;
Experimenting with vegetarian meals;
Considering food combinations in the preparation of meals;
Using nutritional supplements such as brewer's yeast, lecithin, wheat germ, and kelp;
Inventing new recipes;
Discovering new cookbooks;

Juicing vegetables and fruits;
Doing new tricks with old foods;
And so on . . .

Such is the stuff of positive nourishment. Consider what you have to gain from such an approach. It might be good to look over those eight points in managing the transition again—they really are important.

Good luck on your journey into positive nourishment. You'll notice the difference!

NUTRITION AS THERAPY

What we have been talking about so far is what is known as the *maintenance diet*. It is the diet you use over the long term to maintain the balance of all the body systems, selecting food imparting the highest energy, and avoiding food and chemicals of low or no energy and of high toxicity.

What I would like to focus on now are therapeutic diets. These are for temporary use, and are mainly to correct imbalances which have developed in body systems and to eliminate toxins which have built up in the body.

The Orthodox View

In traditional medical practice, the dietary information presented to patients has largely been limited to the four food groups and the MDR's of vitamins and minerals, with virtually no consideration of such things as the energy potential or freshness of food, or the presence of toxic substances in it. As people have become more aware through reading and listening, they have learned that it is difficult to get answers to nutritional questions in a doctor's office, and they are turning elsewhere for those answers.

Doctors have focused attention on areas which they perceive as related to certain diseases or symptom patterns. These include gastric hyperacidity and peptic ulcer (bland diet), heart and blood vessel disease (low-cholesterol diet), gout (low-purine diet), kidney stones (acid or alkaline-ash diet), diabetes (low-carbohydrate diet), overweight (low-calorie diet), diverticulitis (low-roughage diet), and a few others. The value of several of these, even in the areas specified, has been called into question in recent years.

The Holistic View

The holistic approach to nutrition, as to other aspects of life, is to consider the whole individual, not just a symptom. When ill health develops, the holistic assumption is that a balance or set of balances has been disturbed, and that some of the factors involved may be foods low in energy and high in toxic substances, especially if excessive quantities are being consumed. The interaction of dietary with nondietary imbalances is, of course, always taken into account in planning the rebalancing program. The sharp contrast between the holistic approach and the traditional medical-dietetic approach can readily be seen.

Many Different Paths

Many different schools of thought have arisen as alternatives to the standard American diet. These can generally be classed as holistic because they meet, to some extent, the criteria of restoring body balances and of using foods yielding high energy and low toxicity. Most therapeutic systems tend to be designed according to how one views the processes of assimilation of energy and detoxification.

One system[6] sees 80 percent of all chronic disease as caused by a toxic or malfunctioning bowel, while others cite the consumption of "dead" food,[7, 8] consumption of animal products, formation of mucus,[9, 10] blockage of ki (the Japanese term for the flow of electromagnetic energy through body meridians or paths which correspond to various organs),[11] congenital vitamin deficiency,[12] and so on. All of them work for some people under some conditions. There are many paths.

It may be useful to examine some of these approaches briefly to develop a sense of where they lie in a continuum from the standard American diet (SAD) to the opposite extremes of raw food and fasting diets.

A major concern in developing a therapeutic approach should be the rate and extent of transition as a function of the likelihood of the individual to manage and benefit from that transition. The transition should not be unnecessarily extreme. I am aware that many therapeutic programs fail for just this reason. Only in special circumstances (such as cancer or terminal illness) are extremes appropriate.

Therapeutic diets range from the acceptable to the questionable to the totally unacceptable in the public consciousness. I think that three statements can fairly be made in this regard:

1. Acceptance is more a function of familiarity than effectiveness.
2. A major literacy problem regarding diet exists: Many therapies are based on concepts totally unfamiliar to the disease-oriented public and professionals (for example, healing crises, mucus and catarrh, bowel toxicity, dietary stress factors, ecological mental-illness, etc).
3. What is common and acceptable has been controlled almost totally by the medical and dietetics establishments.

Elimination Diets. One concept which has achieved some popularity is that foods and chemicals can produce maladaptive reactions. The central idea is disarmingly simple, but controversial and provocative: Many common foods and chemicals produce physical and mental illness with a wide range of symptoms which are due to withdrawal from addicting foods, or due to cerebral-allergic reactions. The elimination diets used for control simply exclude offending foods and chemicals, usually after extensive testing.

A very well-known and controversial therapy is the Feingold elimination diet for "hyperactivity."[13, 14] The theory links flavors and colors primarily, as well as some preservatives and other food chemicals, to the adverse reactions associated with hyperactive behavior. There have been numerous studies done on the subject, and controversy continues.

It is important to approach the elimination diet in a holistic framework, which should include elimination of sugar and other refined foods, as well as the inclusion of whole health-building foods. The more one thinks about the diet in this context, the better I suspect the results of adhering to it will be.

Intermediate Approaches. The works of Paavo Airola[15] and Bernard Jensen[16] are examples of nutrition programs moderately far removed from the SAD but not extreme or drastic in variation. Virtually unlimited culinary variety is possible.

The Airola Diet is part of a broader framework of "biological medicine" which also uses supplements, herbs, fasting, and baths in the treatment of nearly sixty illnesses, including common poisons. The program is for maintenance as well as therapy, and is guided by a number of principles. The optimum diet should consist, in order, of: (a.) Nuts, grains and seeds; (b.) vegetables; (c.) fruits. Only natural foods should be eaten, and those mostly in the raw or living state. Poisons and toxins should be avoided, as should excessive protein. Also recommended, in addition to the three basic foods above, are: milk, cold-pressed vegetable oils, honey, brewer's yeast, kelp, wheat germ and fish-liver oils, natural vitamin and mineral supplements. A number of do's and don'ts are included as a part of the program.

The Jensen Program[16, 17] is based on the assertion that "death begins in the colon." The majority of chronic illness is seen as being due to toxins in the bowel and the build-up of catarrh, phlegm, and mucus in the body. Diets which foster the elimination of toxins from the body are used. In the course of therapy, a "healing crisis" occurs, reproducing some of the symptoms of illness en route to becoming well.

Vegetarian Diets. Here is a story which epitomizes vegetarianism: Some years ago, when I first met Dick Gregory, he was in the middle of an extensive fruit juice fast. Anxious to make conversation, I asked him in a fit of naiveté one of those questions that you know is stupid before you finish it: "Brother Greg, if all you do is drink juice, where do you get your protein?" A really funny answer made the whole thing worth it: "You don't have to eat hair to grow hair!"

The point is that no one needs to eat protein—just the constituent amino acids which are abundant in fruits, vegetables, and other foods. The literature on vegetarianism is copious, and you might begin with *Diet for A Small Planet.*[18]

The reasons people eat vegetarian diets range from moral and consciousness issues to health reasons to economics to ecological sensitivity. Three types are common: lacto-ovo-vegetarian (with dairy and eggs), ovo-vegetarian (with eggs), and vegan (no dairy or eggs). Vegetarianism is growing in popularity, and, in many ways, has become a metaphor for wholesome eating. But, as with all food, vegetables must be thoughtfully selected, lovingly prepared, and thankfully eaten for optimum health benefits.

The More Extreme Diets. This is a group of diets furthest removed from the SAD and therefore used by fewer people, although with just as much fervor and conviction.

1. *Macrobiotics* is defined as "the application of Oriental philosophy to the biological and physiological science of nutrition."[19] It was introduced into the west by Michio Kushi and Georges Ohsawa. Two basic principles are fundamental to macrobiotics: the yin-yang principle,* by which foods are balanced according to the degree of their yin or yang character, corresponding to the yin or yang aspects of the person; and the concept of *ki* (*chi* in Chinese), in which electromagnetic energy flows through the body in certain paths called meridians. Thus, by balancing the intake of foods, one can balance the energies of the body. A number of rules make this diet seem restrictive to the average Westerner, but, once the rules are mastered, the diet is varied and tasty.

2. Some observers feel that the reason certain diets have destructive effects is because of foods being consumed in the *wrong combinations.* A corollary is that the more different foods are eaten at one time, the greater the likelihood of wrong combinations.[20, 21, 22, 23, 24] A few examples of food-combining laws are no acids with starches, no proteins with carbohydrates, no fats with proteins, etc.

3. Proponents of *raw food diets* claim that cooking the food results in the loss of nutrients, enzymes, and other factors. Arguments for eating only living food center around the availability of enzymes.[25, 26] Grass is considered to be a complete food. Distinctions between raw and live foods are not always made clear by their proponents.

4. *Fruitarian diets* are based on fruit, said to be the most perfect food. It is claimed to be the easiest food to digest and the least mucus-forming.

5. Finally, we come to *fasting*, the ultimate diet. Approaches range from water fasts to various juice, broth, and herb-tea fasts. During the juice fast, as described by Airola,[27] the elimination of dead and dying cells is speeded up, and the building of new cells is stimulated. At the same time, toxic waste products are

*For further elaboration of this theme, see Chapter 32, "A Bird's-Eye View of Oriental Medicine".

actively eliminated, and a normal metabolic rate and cell oxygenation are restored. Juice therapy provides enzymes, nutrients, and other factors quickly and in the correct balance to the cells.

In these two chapters, I have attempted to bring some order to the somewhat confusing field of nutrition, and to show what is required to achieve a holistic perspective in this vital area. In a part of our life which has been subjected to a great deal of theorizing and experimentation, it is well for us never to forget to use our own intuition and "sensing" when we are deciding what to eat. I'm sure that there is no part of our experience in which this is more important than in our nourishment.

19

Overcoming the Power of Death

SCUDDER H. PARKER

Death is defined in several different ways in our culture. Physical death is technically the cessation of heart activity and breathing; though increasingly, because of the advancing technology of life-support systems, death is also described as the ending of brain-wave activity. Putting the fine points of the discussion aside, physical death means that an acting, responding person becomes merely a body, incapable of human interaction.

Simultaneous with the ending of all physical function is the loss of the presence of a *person.* The person who was our loved one is not "here" any more. We cannot speak, relate, or communicate as once we could with that person. Obviously, it is this "loss" of a person which we generally refer to when we speak of death. It is true that what we have called physical death and the loss of the person do not always directly coincide. At times, we say that someone has "died" before his or her physical death, referring to some radical change in character, or to a period of mental impairment or prolonged unconsciousness. We use the word *loss* before the time of physical death as an analogy to explain our separation from some portion of another's humanness, even though their body continues in existence.

A huge weight of feelings is tied to the physical death and loss of a person. To speak of a person's death is to trigger in people a wide range of emotions, including fearfulness, guilt, anger, grief, resignation, and even relief. Deriving from and intertwined with these feelings are all the theories, religious and secular, about death—what it is, what it means, why it happens, what happens after it, etc. And so a third way of describing death is as a recurring social phenomenon—a category of human experience which is a part of the culture and the social institutions of every human community.

When we describe death as a part of every culture we need to acknowledge that its major component is all the painful feelings which have throughout history been associated with the experience of death. Physical pain is perhaps the most obvious pain often associated with death, but just as powerful in shaping our thinking is the pain caused by the removal of a loved one's presence; the sense of weakness and vulnerability aroused by the prospect of our own death; the fear of the unknown; and the sense of responsibility for a person now gone. These, and many more painful feelings related to the experience of someone dying or the prospect of our own death, all deeply stain our thinking about just what death is and what it means.

So thoroughly do these painful experiences color our perceptions that every assumption we make, and every belief we hold about physical death and the experience of losing someone is shaped by them. As human beings we encounter death not in isolation, but through the whole system of ritual, theory, theology, popular wisdom and convention which pervades the society.

We do not know what death would be like in a healthy society. We do not even know that it would exist at all. It is essential for us, in thinking about death, to have a critical awareness that the assumptions which seem unshakable, the "evidence" which seems irrefutable, and the framework for discussion which may seem to be the obvious one, are all, in fact, shaped by the accumulated pain associated with the experience of physical cessation of activity.

It is my purpose in this essay to outline the route along which a new way of thinking about death might proceed. First I will describe the way feelings about death are used by the oppressive systems of society to instill and perpetuate themselves. Second, I will summarize several pieces of evidence which suggest that the current consensus about the inevitability of death may not be unshakable. And third, I will speak from my own experience as a pastor about the process of releasing the emotional tension surrounding our experience of death and the role this can play in clarifying our thinking about life and death.

THE SOCIAL "USE" OF DEATH

The assumption underlying almost every current way of thinking about death is that it is an inevitable part of human experience. It has happened to every human we know about before they attained their two-hundredth birthday. It appears to happen to all the living things, both plant and animal, in our environment. We don't have any firm basis for assuming that it won't happen to each of us. According to the principles of logic the conclusion that physical death is a "virtual certainty" for us all may be justified, but in the passion with which most people will intellectually defend that inevitability, there is something more than a case carefully reasoned. "Learning about death" is assumed to be a vital part of every child's upbringing, but when encountering deaths we do not just confront the fact of physical death and loss. When a child hears that an aunt has died, he or she has all the pain and confusion of the people around her pressed into her consciousness. In other words, our sense of the inevitability of death is not just a carefully thought-out observation about something that happens to living things. It is a way we are taught to feel about our own existence. The sense of inevitability limits what we consider possible for our lives. It affects the way we think about our own development and "aging"; it limits the kinds of challenges we are willing to take on; it is directly linked to a deep sense of hopelessness we have about our own ability to accomplish what we know to be right and good.

The painful feelings associated with physical death which I mentioned above (e.g., fear of pain, of the unknown, of losing loved ones; feelings of guilt, grief and vulnerability) are thus not simply private responses to the reality or threat of death. They are, like the ring in a bull's nose, the point at which oppressive systems in the society get a hold on us. Every time we do something out of fear or resignation, guilt or embarrassment, it is the pain built into our lives which is being tugged at, rather than our capacity for intelligent, creative response. Oppressive economic and social systems have consistently used everything from blatant brutality to subtle manipulation to coerce people into doing things which they would not freely choose to do. Without the feelings of fear, guilt, and hopelessness instilled in us, in large part by our experience of death, the systems of sexism, classism, racism, etc., would collapse of their own weight, because people who were not afraid, guilty or hopeless would refuse to play either the role of oppressor or victim. Every struggle for justice and liberation has been characterized by a commitment to overcoming the power of death, or the threat of death, to control people. "Give me liberty or give me death," is perhaps the most dramatic statement of a commitment not to be ruled by fear any more, but every liberation movement has had to struggle to build up people's pride and overcome that fear which has been instilled in us all, in order to conduct a successful struggle for change.

In addition to manipulating the fear and guilt, the oppressive systems offer many theories which rationalize, interpret and justify these feelings. People are encouraged to live with the grief and pain, to adjust to it, atone for it, compensate for it, or numb it out, rather than to work it through and overcome it. Large chunks of the human ability to reason and respond creatively to the environment get buried deep under the layers of accumulated pain. Because people have been denied the support and the resources to express and overcome their painful feelings, those feelings begin to take on a life of their own which seems to be beyond the reach of reason and order. People decide that wars must be inevitable, that irrational violence and cruelty are fixed parts of human nature, that there are good people and bad people, that they are "past their prime," that "good guys always lose," that "You can't fight city hall," and so on. The recent return of the death penalty in the United States is an appropriate symbolic statement of a social structure's belief that the final way to maintain social "order" is through the manipulation of pain and fear, rather than through a determined struggle to expand our human intelligence.

Finally, there is a tendency to move beyond a sense of the inevitability of death to an intellectual adjustment to its necessity and even desirability. I am not here referring to the carefully-defined emotional experience of acceptance which Kübler-Ross describes as part of the process of dealing with death in terminally ill people. Such an "acceptance" appears to be a constructive and even healthy emotional state. I am speaking, instead, of the tendency to decide in an abstract way that death is not only inevitable, it is also necessary. I remember talking to a friend once and raising questions about the possibility that the body might have the capacity to regenerate organs as a way of maintaining physical life long past what we now think of as possible. After being pushed on that track for a while, he finally said, "What are you trying to say? We *need* death. I mean, if we didn't have it we'd have old people all over the place and we would be overpopulated. The Social Security system would go bankrupt!" The assumption is that death is needed to clean out the "dead wood" and perform a useful function in maintaining society the way we know it. This kind of accommodation to death serves to confine our thinking to familiar channels, and it severely limits our ability to think creatively about new options for coping with urgent human needs, and for organizing our life together.

I want to make it clear at this point that I do not dismiss all previous thinking about the meaning of death. People have always struggled courageously to hold on to their humanity, their sense of community and the goodness of life. Many writings, poems, pieces of music, and stories of people's courage have been essential to preserving and clarifying our sense of the goodness of life and the power of our courage and love.

It is, however, my belief that all our ways of coping with death and thinking about it are so loaded with pain and have been so tied up with the experience of being exploited and manipulated that they are all laced with confusion as well as with wisdom. I am convinced that if we follow the thread which I have identified as the sense of the inevitability or necessity of death we will find that it is itself consistently spun out of our unresolved fear and grief.

ARE WE BORN TO DIE?

At this point, I want to look briefly at four "pieces of evidence" that physical death may not be a necessary or inevitable part of being human. I state the case in this way deliberately because it is a relatively safe and familiar thing to argue that "death is not the end" or that there is a life beyond death. Although I have much sympathy with these beliefs, my concern is not to deny the importance of death to human experience, but *to overcome the power of death in human experience.* I believe that often, when people argue for the continued existence of the spirit beyond physical death, they do it out of a refusal to take the pain surrounding death seriously.

But that pain is serious, it is real, and it is destructive; it is linked to our oppression and our feelings of powerlessness. Although I have no illusions that these four "pieces of evidence" amount to anything like a convincing case that death is avoidable, I find the notion that it may not be inevitable to be the most powerful available tool for challenging the destructive power of the idea that we are "born to die."*

The first piece of evidence that death is not inevitable is simply that we have to be educated to the notion of our own mortality. Young people do not believe that they are going to die. Even quite a few of us who are adults will admit that we don't really believe it at some level of our being. Of course, it has always been assumed that this is a problem of the ego, a blind spot that has to be educated out of us. It would be arrogant and brash to consider yourself worthy of living forever, wouldn't it? And don't we all have a sense that "this isn't right" at one time or another when someone we love dies? My point is simply that we have assumed that such notions are just a sign of our confusion or willfulness, but perhaps they are at least as intelligent as the carefully worded justifications or the busy pretending we were offered as children.

The second piece of evidence is the discovery that our perceptions of reality are shaped by the dimensions through which we experience it. Space and time on planet earth shape our notions about lifespan, aging, and what constitutes reality. But our capacity to project ourselves in imagination and in fact away from this planet, out of this solar system, even out of this galaxy, raises the possibility that there may be unimagined modes of existence available to us. Here, the field of science fiction serves as the tool by which we come to terms with seemingly wild new possibilities.

The third item I would raise as a challenge to our thinking about the inevitability of death is the accumulating evidence that the boundaries between life and death are not so sharp and final as they have appeared to be. I am not sure what is happening in our collective psyche, or the spirit of humankind, but it appears that the kind of separation that death has meant for people over

---

*I gratefully acknowledge here the substantial role which the thinking of Harvey Jackins has played in the development of these ideas. In particular, he first stated clearly for me the possibility that death may not be necessary, and outlined the idea that individual death is no longer necessary to human evolution.

the period of human history may not be necessary or inevitable. Accounts of people who have died and "come back" and of people who have been visited by the spirits of individuals considered dead described by those whose credibility cannot easily be doubted indicates that there may indeed be ways in which the spirits of people who are considered dead are very much present with us. Certainly, such accounts can be used, as I suggested above, in arguing for the unimportance of death. I believe they may also be an indication that the sense of death's inevitability has the power to blind us to dimensions of reality which could be available to us here and now.

The fourth piece of evidence has to do with the process of evolution. The development of new adjustments to the environment, in both plant and animal species, has, until this point in history, relied upon the death of old individuals to make way for the new. There has been no way of communicating a creative adaptation in a species to the other individuals of that species. If individuals did not die, progress could not be made. Death of the individual, therefore, played a very important role in ensuring the survival of the species. There is, however, every indication that arguments from this logic applied to life in the human community are not simply inappropriate, but are tremendously destructive. It is increasingly clear that human society moves forward not by genetic adaptation, but by the exercise of intelligence, planning, and cooperation. The creation and recreation of social organizations and institutions determine survival or nonsurvival for humans. It is possible for humans to communicate accumulated information through culture, speech, and writing, and we have the capacity of assimilating new information and suiting our responses to new situations. Although we may feel skeptical at times about the ability of humans to use our wonderful capacity to adapt and create, it is clear that the age-old function of individual death is not really essential to the survival of our species. We sometimes hear people say, "Well, I'm old, I'm set in my ways. I've got to get out of the way so you young folks can make progress." God forbid that we should take such talk seriously, even though precisely those people may have rigidly insisted on some things that are not helpful. They are really asking for the love, support, and attention we all need to keep thinking and growing in the present.

WORKING THROUGH THE PAIN

I suggested earlier that individuals and institutions in society *could* choose to help people recover from the pain they experience in relation to death rather than manipulate, rationalize, and increase that pain. I am convinced, after eleven years in the parish ministry, that people are really searching for precisely the kind of loving support and attention which will allow them to feel and release the pain stored up in them. What is wanted is not someone who will give answers to questions, but a community to help people work through their grief and fear and to challenge them to start thinking clearly and acting powerfully in the world. And so, with people who are dying, I simply try to be a close and loving friend with whom it is safe to express the anger, the physical pain, the fear, and the grief. I encourage the family to do the same, and often take time, sometimes with the family and always with other friends of mine, to express my own feelings. I try to maintain my relationship with the dying person, even during times of unconsciousness, by assuming there is a conscious being present. Physical affection and humor are essential to create the required closeness and safety. Prayer is often a way in which people who are ill, and their families as well, feel safer expressing deep feelings than just bringing them into conversation.

When dealing with feelings about someone who has died, I continue to learn how people are taught to avoid expressing the grief and anger they feel in response to death. I would like to offer three brief examples of how the pain is internalized and carried with us like a piece of gravel in our knee, rather than exposed and fully expressed so that healing can be complete.

First, there is what I call the "Be polite with God" syndrome. I have talked with many people, who, years after the death of a loved one, begin to redden around the eyes when remembering the deceased. With loving attention and encouragement, the tears will often come with a rush. Almost immediately, they will state the reasoning that has held the grief in place for so long: "I don't know why I'm doing this. I should have been over this long ago. I know it's according to God's will, and I should be grateful for what I have. I try to hold onto my faith and be cheerful, but sometimes I get so depressed." The assumption is that religion is a process of protecting God from our real feelings, and, by an heroic act of will, we are to hold to a rather bleak resolve to stay cheerful and keep a stiff upper lip. For people who do not express themselves in religious terms, the same pattern of denial may express itself in the fear that they are going crazy or "losing control." In others who have buried the grief deeply, there may be an opposite but related fear that they are incapable of feeling the grief any more.

Another reason why people hold onto the grief about losing a loved one is the belief that this is the only way they can hold on to the memory. A kind of nursing and cherishing of the grief takes place. The feeling is that "I don't have the person any more, and so, if I go ahead and cry and grieve and release the pain, there will be nothing left." In fact, what will be left is a clear-eyed, alert human being who can see the world better, who can remember the loved one more clearly, and who can continue working out the relationship to the one who has died more honestly and faithfully. All there is to lose is the pain. And losing the pain helps to regain love for the person lost. It helps one to rediscover one's own energy and delight in the gift of life. People who do allow themselves to go through the grieving invariably resume the business of living more fully and come to realize that the only appropriate, long-term response to the experience of another's death is to be more completely alive in the present.

I was once about to start a funeral when the widow began to talk very loudly and agitatedly. Members of her family rushed up to her and started worrying out loud that she was having one of her "spells." I went over to her and simply asked if she was feeling sad about her husband's death. She burst into tears, and I told her children not to worry about her, but simply to love and support her and to cry with her if they wanted to. The "spell" immediately subsided, and the funeral proceeded with everyone crying beautifully through it. It was clear that these "spells" were the best substitute the woman could find for doing the crying she needed to do. What often happens is that we are forced to substitute a "spell," some kind of medication, some busy activity, or conversation about the weather for the grieving we need to do. It is this kind of substitution which keeps us from really facing our feelings, and which helps instill a broader and more general anxiety and fear about death in us. We weren't really there while it was happening; our emotions, our energies, and our attention were somehow focused somewhere else.

The goal for me in the time I spend with a grieving family is simply to help them to remember as many details about the person as possible—what was good, what was insufferable, what was funny or outrageous, what was difficult about being with him or her and what was wonderful. As people recall these details, bring them back into the present, and respond to them with appropriate feelings, they relate to the experience of death more clearly. There is less need to theorize, to theologize, and to "explain." When the bereaved go through this kind of experience, the fear of death and the oppressive sense of death as a cancer eating away at the present begins to shake loose. People begin to offer their own clear and brilliant thinking about the person who has died, about themselves, and about what is important in their lives. They are then able to reach out and comfort and nurture one another, and to think clearly about just what support each person needs to go through the time of grieving creatively, and to take the next step forward in their lives.

Whenever this is allowed to happen, the fear of death begins to lose its power as a mechanism for social control. Instead of giving up on life and on themselves people are enabled to find new energy and intelligence. We each needs to put our insight and sensitivity to work in our families, workplaces, and communities to assist one another in recovering from the grief, fear and anger we feel.

Although I have spoken a great deal about the question of whether or not death is inevitable, I hope it is clear that my primary concern is not to engage in a debate about whether or not it is inevitable. I simply do not know whether it is or isn't. But if we insist on following that thread which is the theme in human experience that "we are born to die," it will lead us to all the unresolved pain of our own and previous generations. If we allow ourselves to feel and release that pain, we will find that our assumptions about what can't be changed in ourselves, will yield to the power of our love and the creativity of our intelligence. And who knows what the world will look like when that happens?

20

Beyond Death

T. EDWARD ROSS II

T he realms which lie beyond death have held a fascination for imaginative writers throughout the ages, and have produced in people a host of other emotions and attitudes, among them fear, apprehension, curiosity, anxiety, and anticipation. But, in the past few decades, a new element has entered the picture—the personal experiences of a number of people, from all walks of life and from all parts of the globe. At first just a trickle, the accounts of these experiences do not yet constitute a flood, but certainly a robust stream is now flowing as people become a little more comfortable sharing their experiences. Consider the following account:

Two researchers complete a telephone call and note the time. It is 12:15 P.M. They have asked and received permission from the woman at the other end of the line, fifty miles away, to proceed with the experiment. The man begins, "In the name, with the power and by the word—" His co-researcher follows the affirmation silently, timing its preplanned stages with a pendulum held lightly between thumb and forefinger and noting the cessation of its swing at the end of each segment of the request. In less than five minutes, the experiment is concluded and the details entered in a log.

The report, when it comes, is intriguing. "Suddenly," the housewife writes, "the room became excessively cold, and remained so for several minutes. Then came a burst of warmth. It was like a summer breeze, comforting and relaxing. I attributed it to the source of all the other unusual events and paid little heed to it. Then Lew called. He said, 'The house is clear now.' I asked him if it had been cleared at 12:15. He checked, and the answer was yes."

The multiple apparitions, the rapid changes in temperature, the strange sounds had abruptly stopped, and the 200-year-old house was at peace. More importantly, as far as the researchers were concerned, was the implication that two earth-bound souls had been released from their self-made prison, and had been freed to pursue their ongoing journey to a realm of activity and purpose.[1]

RESEARCH INTO LIFE-AFTER-DEATH EXPERIENCES

Like a half-finished sketch, the realm we have glimpsed is slowly being illuminated by the ancient religious lore of the world, and by the scientific work being carried on today. Such researchers as Dr. Elisabeth Kübler-Ross, the Swiss-born neuropsychiatrist; Dr. Karlis Osis, psychologist and one-time director of research for the American Society for Psychical Research; Dr. Russell Noyes, professor of psychiatry at the University of Iowa College of Medicine; and Dr. Raymond A. Moody, Jr., a former professor of philosophy with a degree in medicine, to name a few, have been prominent in this field. They have contributed to a growing body of literature, some published in medical and other professional journals, some for public consumption. Much of the work appears not only to confirm ancient Scriptural statements about the hereafter, but also provides evidence tending toward a single view, detailed and vivid, of the plane beyond death and the pattern of existence in it.

Many who have met with the ravages and shock of severe disease or accident have lost all vital signs—have become clinically dead by the standards of the attending physicians—yet have returned to life and *recalled the experience.*

"I remember hearing the X-ray machine click," relates one such victim, himself a physician, "and that's the last thing I remembered until the early morning of December 24 (five days later) when a nurse came into my room and said, 'Good to have you back with us.' " This man, now a practicing psychiatrist, was then in the wartime army. He was pronounced dead not once, but twice, at times nine minutes apart, on December 21. Any trained rescue-squad member will tell you that the human brain cannot function more than three or four minutes without oxygen. Altogether, this man survived for nine minutes without breathing. An orderly noticed some movement, but he was examined and again pronounced dead. As a last resort, adrenalin was injected into his heart, and eventually, three days later, he regained consciousness.

What concerns us here is his memory of what transpired in the nine minutes while he was clinically dead, for it is an account of a pattern that is substantiated in similar cases over and over again—different in minor details, but identical in overall design. Our young doctor-to-be 'awoke,' sat up, and *saw his body lying on the bed.* He then 'walked' from the room and endeavored to locate the ward attendant. To his horror, he was unable to do so; they stood face to face, and then walked *through each other.*

Despite the mental shock of these events, he nevertheless held one goal uppermost in his mind—to catch the train to the city where he was to enter medical school. In rapid succession, he found himself outside the building, traveling over the terrain at great speed, and noting, as one would from a low-flying plane, a river and a town, to which he dropped down. A man he questioned simply didn't respond. He leaned against the guy-wire of a telephone booth to think things over, and discovered that it passed right through his body. Frantic, he felt the need of the body that he had left at the hospital. It occurred to him that the medical officer might be working on it, preparing it for the morgue!

No sooner had he made the decision to return than he was back in the building, searching for himself. He began to look for his fraternity ring. Lying in an isolated room was a body half covered with a blanket. A hand lay outside, and, on a finger, he recognized the ring. He could not communicate with the attendants he saw, and he could not reenter his body.

Desperate, he became aware of a growing brightness. The walls disappeared and were replaced, as in a film, by a panoramic view of all he had done in his life. Out of the light, a form appeared. He identified it as a male, and it was filled with power and compassion. All his fear was gone. Many other scenes appeared in sequence, and finally he saw an altogether different realm filled with music, technical invention, and study, where the people and buildings seemed structured of brilliant light. The bond of attraction to the being, who appeared inextricably joined to these visions, began to loosen. He became conscious and aware that he was in his own body. It was the morning of December 24.[2]

The importance of this account is not so much that in later years he was to see in a magazine scenes he had visited in his out-of-body state, or that his goals as a doctor were to be greatly changed by the episode. The real meaning for us lies in the recollection of an experience which is common to some others declared clinically dead who have survived to recount a similar pattern of "location" and "event."

Are such experiences caused by hallucination stemming from illness or drugs? Dr. Karlis Osis has analyzed over 800 professional reports of this kind and believes the pattern that emerges is consistent with the survival of consciousness. There are so many accounts so unified in their content that it begins to seem reasonable to credit this kind of 'unscientific' explanation, based on "anecdote."

Here are samples of statements taken from Dr. Raymond A. Moody's fifty interviews with those who had nearly encountered death: "Floating in a dark space" (after a near-fatal head injury); "Peace, comfort, ease" (after a heart attack); meeting with deceased relatives and friends viewed as "helpers"; a "brilliant light" associated with a being of definite personality who is at times both conversational and telepathic; weightlessness and freedom of movement; a body of vaporous substance that nevertheless conforms in rough outline to the physical body; heightened mental acuity, but inability to see oneself in a mirror.[3]

A similarity pervades these reports, each of which corroborates the next. They are indicative of what all the world's religions have sought to convey in greater or lesser degree, but fall short of any test or "proof," which the scientific mind requires.

Several centers in the United States have had an interest in collecting these fascinating data. The Division of Parapsychology of the University of Virginia Medical School, the Stanford Research Institute in Palo Alto, and the Cancer Institute of the University of California, to name but a few, have taken an active interest in the subject, while the Association for Transpersonal Psychology has members who are individually concerned. The Theta Project of the Psychical Research Foundation at Durham, North Carolina, is a worldwide program involving people with scientific training, people who expect to die soon, and project volunteers. While the main thrust of the program is the study and counselling of the terminally ill, the exploration of death naturally examines the continuation of consciousness as well.

Academic interest is today being paralleled by popular writings, some of them of a high order. An example is a best-seller[4] based on the tragic crash of an airliner in the Florida Everglades and the subsequent reappearance of its captain and flight engineer on various scheduled flights long after they had perished in the accident. A "rescue mission" was later performed by sensitives who apparently succeeded in bringing awareness of their demise to the crew members and assisting them to find their way to another dimension.

This theme was carried forward by the same author in a well-researched book on the R-101 dirigible disaster which took place in France in 1930. Forty-eight of the passengers and crew lost their lives when the giant dirigible that was intended to revolutionize air travel crashed into the French countryside, after being buffeted by wind and rain, on its maiden voyage to India.

The material in this case differs from that compiled by the medical researchers in that it was received through an intermediary source, a medium. Sir Arthur Conan Doyle was then still living and was at the center of a group of military officers, businessmen, and scientists who researched the case, including such names as Sir William Barrett, the physicist from the University of Dublin, and Dr. Julian Huxley, the noted Oxford biologist. The catalyst for their research was the celebrated medium and clairvoyant, Eileen Garrett, founder of the Parapsychology Foundation, who worked with many prominent American and European literary and scientific figures of the day. Despite exhaustive testing by scientists in many world-renowned centers, the explanation of her ability to enter a trance state and contact those who lost their lives in the accident was not discovered. The enormous weight of technical detail which she eventually amassed not only explained the reasons for the disaster, but went far in outlining the condition of those cut off from earthly existence.

Flight Lieutenant Irwin, in command of the airship, was one of a half-dozen persons who "reported" through Eileen Garrett and other sensitives the details of the crash. Of the fifty-three technical points received from an entity who gave every sign of being Captain Irwin, military and government experts concluded that at least forty-five were authentic and accurate communications. Nearly all were points which Mrs. Garrett could not possibly have known, such was their technical nature.

Even more significant than the technical explanations was the clear-cut description of the transition of those who died in shock. They were men of competence, with balanced interests and superior technical skills; for example, Captain Irwin was a former Olympic athlete and a man of long experience and proven ability. Their voices came through the medium, with all the characteristics by which their friends had known them, even to grammatical usage and personal touches of humor, and their sense of duty and urgent motivation ran through the communications like a unifying thread.

THE REALM OF AFTER-LIFE

The realm that emerges from these carefully recorded sessions with Eileen Garrett resembles in many respects the life that we know here. Even though the pilot was conscious of facing death several hours beforehand, the change from the physical body had occurred in moments and without pain. He nevertheless states that the first obstacle to overcome is incomplete awareness of the fact of death.

So alike did he find the states of life and after-life that, without preparation, he felt the change might not in every case be noticeable. There was nothing ethereal or heavenly about it. He found himself in a grey, damp, barren region "like the wastes of Belgium I used to fly over." Many people could linger there for years, he said.

As on earth, when he was in an unenviable state, he determined to get out of it, and, with that decision, began to succeed. The brighter realms, he learned, were accessible only to those who had passed through a refining process that permitted them entry. Though he found no physical suffering, the potential for mental duress was very great, due to one's increased awareness and sensitivity. All on earth, he said, should realize that, as they have lived and worked, so will their awareness be in the hereafter, that it is an ongoing process, and that we are forever creating our own level of attainment.

In another remarkable account written in 1969 by an English author,[5] contact with this other realm is carried a step further. Based on her personal sense of the presence of a close friend who had died of cancer, a former Anglican nun, teacher, and psychologist, she develops a lengthy description of the hereafter in simple, yet vivid terms. Careful to say that the book was not a product of automatic writing, she nevertheless considers it "a composite effort," the result of "tuned minds" and telepathy.

The return to consciousness after death, she notes, is "overwhelming." The first task is to look at a "movie" of one's life "for comparison with its original plan." Although life is a matter of progressing consciousness, "the minute after you die, you will be exactly the same in heaven." Heaven, it appears, is no super-welfare state, and one has to earn every step of progress one makes.

There are "receiving stations" staffed by volunteers to ease the transition. Since thought is immediately creative, the means exist to adjust the surroundings to fit the needs of the new arrival. For one who dies of wounds or injuries, a nursing ward exists; for one who is prepared for a peaceful change, there is a garden. At first, communication is with words, then by mental exchange. Along with weightlessness, there is an element of timelessness. Although it may be very gradual, progress is made toward creative activity.

Always, there is help if it is sought. Helpers at the receiving stations consist of volunteers who learn from their dedication—for them it is a journey into reality. Prayers from earth are meaningful, for those who have recently died respond quickly to the vibrations of the ones to whom they were close.

Communication from this realm, the author implies, may be by telepathy, activated by the desire to penetrate the barrier of density that surrounds our earthly life, or it may be arranged from "stations" in the other plane by volunteers and specialists who have understanding of the forces involved.

"Rescue missions" may also be performed from the earth plane, to persuade and escort an earthbound soul—one who cannot or will not make the passage on his own. Such souls appear to link themselves to this plane to their own detriment, held back by the attractions or involvements of the life just left behind. Explicit warning is given to those who would attempt such work, that they, in the words of Mrs. Greaves, our English author, "must be very pure in heart and very sure of divine assistance."

ULTRA-SENSING

One final avenue of exploration remains to be discussed, that of *ultra-sensing*, through which all that we have gleaned seems to be confirmed and upheld.[6] Ultra-sensing is what dowsers do when they seek and locate targets that are beyond the horizon of the five senses, whether water, gas, oil, missing persons, or archaeological artifacts. Those who sense in this way are true psychics, and pass beyond the limitations of space to find what they want.

The new-old ability of ultra-sensing lies within us all. It has regularly been substantiated in recent years in many types of cases, the incident presented in the opening paragraphs being one example. The researchers in that instance were never closer to the target zone than fifty miles, yet were sufficiently aware of what was taking place there to act efficiently and successfully in the owner's behalf.

There has been a step-by-step evolution in the art of ultra-sensing. When this vibratory rate is achieved by the individual, he or she has acquired the protection necessary to enable attempting the kind of rescue mission described. An indication of what is involved follows, to show what must take place before fear of the unknown can be banished.

The ultra-sentient practitioner properly begins an approach to the earth-bound entity with permission. A surprising number of us have had encounters of the kind met with by the housewife. What was unusual was her determination to seek help and find a remedy. Without it, the research team could not have successfully worked with her to bring an end to the haunting, and, presumably, to effect a rescue mission as well. It was the *request* that initiated the attempt, and that is assumed to be the first step.

The next step is for the practitioner to determine his own ability vis á vis the case at hand. May I? Can I? Then, should I? Is this the appropriate moment? One learns to trust the answers one receives from these rapid, preparatory, inward probings. When satisfied on all counts, one goes to the target site, whether next door or a thousand miles away, where the earth-bound soul is seen as a shadowy image. At this point, the figure may be addressed or referred to a higher being or beings to await the results. If the choice is to go ahead, much the more arduous way, the practitioner must then explain to the entity, "I come to assist, to give peace and purpose, and to escort you to the realm for which you are destined, and where friends and relatives wait to extend a welcome."

The entity is seen as male or female in general appearance and attitude. In all but the rare cases in which an obsession governs an entity, there is a more or less willing acquiescence. Fear may be present, but will not deter the earth-bound soul from accompanying the rescuer through the astral darkness. The "reception committee," referred to also by mediums and returnees from clinical death, is waiting, and consists of either two or three personages. They first appear as pinpoints of light; as they grow larger, recognizable faces may appear. The soul-entity then seems to vanish into these points of light, and the rescuer is left to make his return and to give thanks.

This regime has been followed in recent years with increasing confidence, as many can testify. It is both repeatable and, to the qualified candidate, teachable. Success is partly measurable in an objective sense—heavy footsteps cease, odd sounds are no longer heard, pets resume normal habits of sleep, and so on. Success in a subjective sense is complete. The home, office, or hospital room is "seen" in an altogether different light. A benign and welcoming atmosphere replaces the unpleasant and hostile emanations immediately. Of all the possible effects, most interesting are those related to health. Illness is known to abate or remit in many instances. This accords with ancient precedent, and is consistent with what has been outlined of the pattern beyond death.

Let us then close this brief introduction to the subject with a quotation and a question. In his great soliloquy, Hamlet refers to the "bourne from which no traveler returns"—good poetry, certainly, but not, it now seems, in accord with observation. We do travel, we do return—and we remember. If we can know where we are heading after we leave this plane, we will be better prepared to live there. Might we not, also, be better prepared to live in the here and now?

PART IV
Restoring Health and Wholeness in Ourselves and Others

21

The "Breakdown Lane"

PETER ALBRIGHT

This section of our book deals more directly with issues relating to ill health than any other part of the book. To define illness as ill health or health breakdown—that is, in terms of health—always points to the goal of return to health. This is good mental programming.

This complete spéctrum of health and health breakdown is one which I have adapted from a similar definition of health and disease; I am unable to locate the source. I think that a graphic depiction of the spectrum is very helpful in our consideration of health breakdown. It is shown in Figure 1.

I often use the language of the interstates and motorways when I think of this diagram and the concept it represents. In those terms, the left half of the diagram is the travel lane, and the right half is the breakdown lane, where repairs must be made before one may reenter the travel lane and zoom away!

The breakdown lane is the usual domain of traditional medicine, and doctors and nurses are generally in charge of what is going on. The goal of their activity is to deal with a patient who is mildly, seriously, or critically ill, and to transport that person safely across the line into the healthy space, quite often into the barely symptom-free area. There, other people, such as families and home health nurses, are expected to assume the majority of the responsibility for further recovery. Such things as diet, vitamins and other supplements, and alternative methods of healing are outside the sphere of interest and expertise of many, if not most, medical practitioners.

The travel lane is the usual domain of holistic health care. There, the person (client, patient) is in charge of things, and may be helped by one or more practitioners of his choice. The goal of

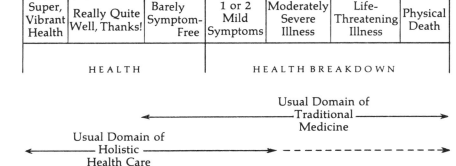

Figure 1. Spectrum of Health and Health Breakdown

their work together is to see that the person remains as vibrantly healthy as possible. If health proves hard to maintain and the person slips across the line into the one-or-two mild symptoms category, they will labor together with perhaps a bit more vigor to return her to the healthy area, of course as close to vibrant health as possible.

Of special note is the section of the holistic health line which is broken into dashes. This includes people who relate primarily to holistic health care and who become seriously ill. In the area of the dashes, their practitioners maintain active concern about them, and will, if possible, continue therapy, although they clearly recognize that specialists in the treatment of severe or advanced health breakdown are in charge at the moment.

In the center of the diagram there is an obvious overlapping of the areas of traditional medicine and holistic health care. In this overlapping area, a person can most clearly benefit from either or both types of care. One might also think of drawing dashes on the traditional medicine line clear to the vibrant end of the healthy territory. That will certainly be appropriate when enough traditional practitioners also practice holistic health care, but, at the moment, there are far too few to make the dashes realistic!

In terms of our book, the activities of the previous section on creating and maintaining health and wholeness technically belong to the righthand side of the diagram, although it is obvious that people in any of the stages and situations described there may be at one time or another in a state of health breakdown, even to the point of serious illness or death. Similarly, while the activities of this section belong in a discussion of health breakdown, it is clear that most of its chapters discuss things which are also useful in maintaining health, right up to the vibrant level.

What is the significance of health breakdown? It is easy to look at a person with pneumonia and conclude that the situation is "caused by" the staphylococcus germ or the pneumococcus germ, especially since a selected antibiotic drug may result in the clearing of symptoms, and often in a barely symptom-free state. What more and more investigators into the subject of health are finding is that health breakdown on the physical plane is but the outer manifestation of imbalance or imbalances at the deeper mental, emotional, and spiritual levels of being.

This does not mean that the antibiotic must not be used when the health breakdown is at the stage where life or tissue and organ preservation is at stake. It is a rash person indeed who would deny another person the benefits of modern treatment for a severe health breakdown—that is the time when such treatment *must* be used.

What is important is to realize that the breakdown itself reflects imbalance at a deeper level. Before, during, and after health breakdown, therapy can be directed at the deeper levels with great benefit to the suffering person. In England, for instance, it is not uncommon for a healer (other than the doctor) of the patient's or doctor's choice to enter the patient's hospital room when he is seriously ill and perform any one of a number of alternative healing techniques. In the United States, only the clergy presently enjoy this privilege.

Similarly, as noted in our discussion of cancer, modes of therapy affecting deeper levels of being are very successfully used in conjunction with standard orthodox therapy. As the results of combined therapies become more widely known, it can be predicted with safety that their benefits will be appreciated by more and more afflicted people.

The many articles in this section, while they by no means constitute a catalogue of therapies, focus attention on the subtler energies of our bodies and how they can be influenced by subtle means, resulting in notable changes on the physical level. In the next chapter, for example, Dr. Oscar L. Morphis, a distinguished cancer therapist, shares his unusual insights into critical energies of the human organism, and how unhealthy patterns can be turned into healthy patterns at deeper levels of being. Late in the section is a brief view of orthodox (traditional, allopathic) medicine, which will continue to hold an undeniably important place in the management of health breakdown.

22

The Miracle of In-Cell-Igence

OSCAR L. MORPHIS

T his chapter is intended to direct the reader's attention to some ideas about the nature of human cells and tissues which I think help to explain why we are either in a state of health or in a state of health breakdown. I would also like to cite some of my clinical experience in the field of cancer therapy and to relate my reflections about health and breakdown to what I have been observing for a number of years in clinical practice.

First, let's talk a bit about some of the things that are known scientifically about us as human beings and about our natural world. It is known that only when *vibration* occurs is it possible for us to *sense* with the five sensing organs, the eyes (light), ears (sound), tongue (taste), nose (odor), and skin (touch).

THE IMPORTANCE OF VIBRATION

What is *vibration* and what is its effect? All vibration is the result of movement of electric charges or wave forms. It is this movement which our sensing devices detect. Electromagnetic waves (including light waves) travel at 186,400 miles per second. The *visible* part of the electromagnetic spectrum is only one octave of the spectrum; many other octaves cannot be sensed by the eyes. The highly efficient ear can detect about seven octaves of the sound spectrum, but there are many more octaves in the sound spectrum which the healthy ear cannot hear. Sound waves travel at about 1,050 feet per second. The eyes and ears together sense about 95 percent of the stimulation detected by the five physical senses.

However, our combined five senses perceive *far less than 1 percent* of the ocean of wave forms and vibrations in which we live! Therefore, no one can possibly expect to see, hear, taste, smell, or feel more than a tiny part of the stimulation which is reaching our bodies from outside sources.

All matter is in a state of vibration at all times; what are actually vibrating are minute energized particles, or bits of energy. Let us use water as an example of this. Water is made up of atoms of hydrogen and oxygen in a certain ratio. Under the conditions in which water is in the liquid state, there are just so many atoms per cubic inch or centimeter; thus, water is said to have a certain density in the liquid state. It will run through our fingers.

If we then heat water until it becomes steam, the main change it undergoes is that the particles spread out, and the water becomes less dense. We can pass our hands right through steam. Conversely, when water is cooled, the particles come much closer together, and the water becomes solid, forming ice, which can be held in the hand. All of the "solid" objects with which we are familiar, such as our houses, cars, furniture, and our bodies are simply energized particles in a state of constant vibration, held very closely together in a relatively dense form.

INTERFERENCE PATTERNS

One of the more familiar examples of vibration is obtained by dropping a pebble into a pool of water. We all know the concentric circles which radiate out from the spot where the pebble entered the water. This is a very good example to use because it illustrates an extremely important phenomenon for our discussion—namely, interference patterns. Suppose that, instead of dropping just one pebble into the pool, we drop two pebbles simultaneously and near each other. At the time the outer circle from one pebble encounters the outer circle from the other pebble, a totally new pattern emerges, known as an interference pattern. These patterns are neither necessarily good or bad; they are merely new. The purpose of introducing interference patterns into our discussion is that, as we shall see, they may play an extremely important part in the life of living cells.

A more complicated example of interference patterns, and a fascinating one, is a *hologram*. A hologram is made by exposing photographic film to laser light which has been split into two beams by passing it through semitransparent, or one-way, glass. The two beams are thus somewhat out of phase when they are allowed to fall on a three-dimensional object. The resulting image is recorded on the photographic film. When similar laser light is thrown on the film, the viewer sees what appears to be the original three-dimensional object *behind* the film! The image looks real; it looks solid enough to touch or to pick up. But it cannot be sensed by touch; the hand would pass right through the space where it appears to be.

The hologram is not a picture. It is a frozen moment of the composite wave-pattern in the room, captured in a light-sensitive emulsion. This emulsion (film), if viewed by ordinary light, would appear clear. If, however, it is viewed by coherent (laser) light with characteristics similar to the original light, the image will be "reconstructed" in all its dimensions.

Since every part of the film contains all of the information, even a tiny piece of the film can reproduce the entire image! It is not the film which reconstructs the image; it is the light that does it by striking the interference pattern.

STRUCTURE FORMED BY VIBRATION

The hologram illustrates how light images can be created by interference patterns. Another example shows how mass particles can actually be moved and distributed by sound vibrations, showing how structure is formed by vibratory energy.

In this experiment, first elaborated on by Dr. Hanns Jenny, sand particles are spread out over the surface of a thin metal plate which is then bombarded by coherent sound vibrations of a single frequency and amplitude. The sand vibrates and collects into nodal patterns. As long as the frequency and amplitude of the sound and the shape of the plate are kept exactly the same, the nodal pattern is faithfully reproduced. If any of the factors are changed, however, the nodal pattern is altered; its structure is changed. If a second frequency is introduced, a new pattern is produced. If more frequencies are added, these result in more complicated forms.

Many frequencies, amplitudes, and modulations produce a symphony of sounds, which, in turn, produce a structure composed of physical particles arranged in certain geometric configurations (tetrahedrons and quadrahedrons, such as are found throughout nature). All these factors must be in perfect harmony, or a chaotic arrangement of the physical particles will result.

This process is a lot like the symphony orchestra, which must perform in perfect harmony to sound exactly right. If one instrument hits a wrong note, a frequency is altered, changing the interference pattern and spoiling the harmony.

If one could see under a microscope a phonograph record of this wrong note in the otherwise harmonic passage, one would see an actual change in the structural mass of the groove in the record as a result of the altered interference pattern. The phonograph record is a "frozen" interference pattern, just as the emulsion freezes the interference pattern on the holographic film.

INTERFERENCE PATTERNS IN THE CELL

We can now begin to look at the action of interference patterns in living cells and tissues. When vibrational frequency increases to very high levels (10^{40} hertz and up), its energy, if the wave form is concentrated by pressure to high densities, results in the production of *mass*. Mass particles become atoms, molecules, cells, and, finally, tissues. With the additional help of sound frequencies, interference patterns are produced. If the correct harmonies (interference patterns) are produced, the symphony (the cell) is perfect. If any part is out of tune (phase), then discord (disease or imperfection in the cell) is the result. Thus, the cell is a symphony of harmonious interference patterns.

Human beings, like plants and other animals, germinate from a seed. We know that this minute seed must contain the entire blueprint for the growth and development of the adult organism. But this is not really a "blueprint"—it is an interference pattern! I will elaborate on this below.

Another term by which we might know this particular interference pattern is "the kinds of intelligence which reside within the cell." This is a rather cumbersome term, so, to represent it, I have coined another term: In-cell-igence, or *Incelligence*.

As each single cell is produced, it must already contain three basic types of Incelligence. First, it must know if it is a heart cell, a brain cell, or a liver cell. This is individualized Incelligence. Then, it must have group Incelligence, which is the vibrating together of many cells to form an organ. Lastly, it must contain collective Incelligence, to integrate with the entire body as a unit. These three orders correspond to the individual instrument, the violin section, and the entire symphony orchestra.

WHAT CAUSES DISHARMONY?

If all levels of Incelligence are in harmony, the organism is perfect, just as the symphony is perfect if all the instruments are playing correctly. But what causes a perfect organism to become out of tune, to vibrate inharmoniously, to step out of phase? We cannot discover the cause by using strictly the five senses, since the cause is acting at a very subtle level; it is influencing an electrical charge which we cannot sense or identify as such. We can only "sense" the effect, which is the *pressure* (displacement) of the charge, producing wave or anti-wave form.

Inappropriate pressures produce altered interference patterns, which, in turn, produce structural change, such as a change from a normal cell to a cancer cell. The pathologist recognizes this change under the microscope. If this is not corrected, the abnormal cell becomes two abnormal cells, which become four, and this continues until the entire organ is abnormal, and eventually the whole organism is affected.

What kinds of stimulation can produce the very subtle but crucial changes in electrical charge which lead through pressure changes and altered interference patterns to structural change? The kinds of stimulation are basically four: physical, chemical, electrical, and "psychological" (a term in which we might include mental, emotional, and spiritual forces).

The first three of these four are already recognized and generally accepted as being capable of producing discord within cells. It is the fourth, however, which is the least understood and may well turn out to be the most important.

Certainly one of the sites of psychological activity is the brain; there may be others, although this is controversial. The brain works twenty-four hours a day receiving, interpreting, and transmitting wave forms. We receive through our senses (five plus others), interpret through our Incelligence, and act appropriately through our transmission systems, just as Jenny's plate receives energy, vibrates the sand, and forms nodal patterns. If this is altered at the individual, group, or collective levels, the structural pattern is changed.

CHANGING DISCORD TO HARMONY

What can be done by or for a patient, let us say a cancer patient, at this subtle level to begin to "turn the process around"? No matter what else is done, the patient will not get well unless he can again harmonize his individual symphony. He must alter his interpretation of, and reaction to, outside stimuli, for, if he doesn't, he will continue reinforcing the disharmony. Medicine, surgery, or radiation are modalities which modify the altered interference pattern and are applied to synchronize the physiologic state. However, the *thought pattern* must also be corrected to assist in balancing the corrected interference pattern and maintaining that balance.

Since 1971, this hypothesis has been under investigation by Dr. O. Carl Simonton and Stephanie Simonton, with whom I have been associated in practice for the past several years. We have been caring for, treating, and studying patients with advanced cancer who have been referred to us. We have been dealing with two groups of patients. In the first group are people with the following characteristics: They have had the standard therapy for their cancer, including surgery, radiation, chemotherapy, and tender loving care. They have been involved with us in gentle and thorough interviews and discussions, and we have become convinced that these particular people should not be included in the special program described below. The reasons for this are varied, but mostly center around their feelings about the inevitability of death from their disease and the futility of pursuing special programs to try to alter the process.

In the second group are people with the following characteristics: They, too, have already had the standard forms of therapy and management described above. Upon thorough interview and discussion, they appear to have a real interest in exploring alternate possibilities for working with us toward the healing of their bodies. In fact, they can be described as having a strong drive to become well again, and a strong belief that such a thing is possible.

Patients in the second group are invited to enter the special treatment program. This program includes, among other things, extensive counseling about attitudes toward cancer and introduction to a technique of visual imagery, individually designed for each patient, to permit the patient to take an active and real part in the healing of his body.

AN EXCITING DIFFERENCE

When we contrast the two groups, the results are dramatic. All those in the first group have experienced the progression of their disease which is usually predicted, culminating in death. In the second group, a surprising number have been able to turn the process around, not only regaining health, but maintaining that health far beyond known medical expectations. The essence of this has been a change of lifestyle from one of worry, stress and depression to an attitude of optimism and hope which leads to positive action.

Remember, all the medical factors were the same. The major difference between those who died and those who continued to live has been primarily their ability or inability to change psychologically. At first, it was difficult to believe that a human being could actually alter the growth pattern of cancer. When, in addition to good standard medical care, these patients learned to deal with their problems and stresses, body tissues were rebuilt. It was only after we had seen this pattern repeated again and again that we allowed ourselves to believe that what we hoped for was actually true.

Health is a harmonious symphony of Incelligence. A physician's (or other healer's) function is to help patients achieve a balance and maintain it. This cannot be done unless the treatment itself is complete. Along with the physical methods of medicine, surgery, and radiation, the patient with advanced disease has to be helped to think positively, develop goals, discover a reason to live, and claim worthiness to have good health. Once the physician fully understands the entire process of treatment, the physician's own Incelligence will help the patient to reestablish proper interference patterns. The ultimate responsibility, however, remains with the patient, and depends on how much that particular unique person wishes to become whole!

23

Meditation: A New Way of Being

BETS ALBRIGHT

When I was a child, we had a family friend who was a Hindu. He wrote wonderful stories for children, about India, and I considered him a special person. One day, I was roller-skating in Central Park and saw my Indian friend seated upon a very large rock with his face to the sun and his eyes closed. I removed my skates and sat quietly on the grass below the rock and waited. It seemed a long time to an active ten-year-old, but, finally, he opened his eyes—and, when he saw me, smiled and beckoned me to come and sit beside him. Very timidly, I asked him what he had been doing, sensing that it was something outside of my experience.

"I was meditating," he answered.

"Oh," I said, still mystified. "What do you meditate about?"

"I meditate upon the silence that comes between noises," said Mr. Mukerji. He did not say any more, and I was much too shy to ask more—so that was the end of my early education in the art of meditation.

It was not a subject that was much discussed at that time, at least not in the confines of my family and social life. But I did not forget my encounter. At times, particularly during summers when I had the opportunity to be alone in the woods of northern New Hampshire, I would try to imagine what "the silence that comes between noises" was like. Sometimes, I even felt for a brief moment that I had grasped something—but I was unable to hold onto it for any length of time.

Years later, when I became interested in meditation, and when my husband and I took a course in Transcendental Meditation and became regular meditators, I realized that Mr. Mukerji's technique was as satisfactory as my mantra.

Exploring further, Peter and I took a course in Silva Mind Control, and our "alpha thinking" expanded. It is "alpha thinking" that produces slow alpha-wave cycles in the brain and enables us to channel our minds and bodies in positive-creative patterns. We meditated in the sanctuary at the Findhorn Community in northern Scotland, at the Fellowship of the Inner Light at Virginia Beach, in small groups and in large groups, on planes and buses and beaches, on cushions and "seiza" benches, with people of all ages and nationalities, and by ourselves.

We did not become experts at meditation or firm proponents of any one technique. But we did come to understand that meditation is an important "new" dimension of life. New, that is, to most of us in a modern, industrialized society. Meditation did not originate in our western civilization, but it proves to be a good antidote to the stress that our way of life produces.

It is very much more than a sort of spiritual aspirin tablet or cure for symptoms! Meditation, or "alpha thinking," if you prefer, is a way to move from our overused "left-brain," or thinker, to our "right-brain," the creative hemisphere so often neglected in our think-tank oriented way of life.

In his book *How to Meditate*, Lawrence LeShan says that "we work toward a new understanding of a way of being in the world—a new way of relating to reality. We discover long lost parts of ourselves. Our zest, vitality, efficiency, capacity to love and relate increase and deepen. We begin to know that each of us is a part of all others. We come to a new way of perceiving and relating to the world."[1]

In our first flush of enthusiasm for meditation, my husband and I held a class in relaxation and self-healing in which we taught a simple meditation technique. We wanted to bring the benefits of meditation to those who could not afford TM or who were put off by the faintly religious implications of such a technique. Our class was a wonderful experience, but we soon learned the difficulty of trying to fit an assortment of people into one simple "this-is-the-way" scheme!

If people have difficulty with visualization, they need help in finding simple paths down which their minds can wander in comfort and relaxation. A pattern of imagery that may seem terrific to you will be very awkward for another person. I remember a long session of carefully planned guided imagery at a conference I attended. Everything was going well until our leader took us mentally into an all blue garden. My mind balked. I simply could not get with it, and the rest of the session was lost on me! However, most people who are eager to change their thought patterns, to move into altered states of consciousness, and to learn healthier, more effective ways of being in the world, can be helped to find a way of meditating that is right for them.

Swami Rama has said that "meditation is the state of being established in one's own essential nature." In the next chapter, Eileen Noakes of Devon, England, will describe how meditation fits into our body, mind, and spirit concept, and how vital meditation is to the coming of a new age in each of us.

We do not plan to describe in this book the many techniques for meditation which are available for use. Each person who seeks to go within through meditation must personally select the appropriate way or ways. We do not advocate one way, nor do we wish to overlook possible useful methods. We will emphasize primarily the philosophy of meditation and its place in our lives and in the evolution of our society to a higher level of consciousness. We also offer a bibliography which includes excellent books on meditation techniques.

24

Meditation: The Rainbow Bridge

EILEEN NOAKES

editation concerns not only the spiritual but every
aspect of our subtle and complex constitution. It
requires the building of the rainbow bridge be-
tween the lower self and the higher self, and between the higher
self, or soul, and the world of the spirit. This bridge can only be
built on a foundation of alignment of the physical, emotional, and
mental bodies. Therefore, the care and healing of these three
bodies is important. The physical body is just the tip of the iceberg, and to deal with this outer aspect of ourselves without taking
into account our integral relationship with the vast cosmos would
be like trying to melt the iceberg by placing a hot-water bottle on
the tip! It is such a small, and yet such an important, part of the
whole. This is the paradox—the awareness of the importance of
the physical body as a vehicle of Divine individuality on the plane
of matter, combined with the recognition that it is simply the
outer expression of inner forces and conditions.

We only need more light, in the esoteric sense, to be sure of the
existence of the soul, and this light is becoming available. If,
through our meditations, we invoke this light, we shall help to
produce a powerhouse of light on earth which will greatly hasten
the evolution of human consciousness. The result of making soul
contact, of meditating, and of directing energy correctly, will be
intelligent service and the practice of loving living. Meditation is
not just a matter of sitting quietly and listening for inspiration. It
is very much a matter of helping to transform the world. To be effective as an instrument of service, we need to give some thought
to physical and emotional wholeness.

When we have considered healing the personality and clearing the channels, we begin to turn towards meditation. This is not something apart from our daily lives, because eventually the whole of living will become a meditation. Part of what this means is simply a way of paying attention to every experience and being sensitive to life forces. For example, when walking alone in the early morning along a beach below tall cliffs, topped by green undergrowth, with seagulls whirling about and the sun shining through the mist and sparkling on the sea, are we going to immerse ourselves in this experience? Will we be, as the Essenes would say, "communing with the Angel of Joy," flooding ourselves with this beauty, making it part of ourselves? Or will we walk along worrying about some misunderstanding we have to go back and face, or the fact that people are coming to lunch and we do not know what to give them, or the fact that the price of vegetables has gone up? If we are going to worry, we might just as well be sitting at home in a dark cellar. To live vibrantly every moment, really experiencing life every moment, can make the whole of life a form of meditation, and this includes the mundane.

Now, some people worry that meditation is difficult, and wonder if they are ready for it. Well, not everybody is ready. But, when we begin to think about it, this worry is an indication that we are ready. It is a call of the soul. It has been said that when we have exhausted the best that the personality has to offer through the course of many lives, then we turn to meditation.

We are all deeply concerned about a number of things that have happened in the world, and we ask ourselves how we could have done these terrible things which are the result of our greed and insensitivity. But we are not helpless in the face of all these things, however hopeless we may feel. It is tremendously important, in the course of meditation, either alone or with others, to lift these situations into the Light. This is a very important service to be performed, because situations can be transformed by bringing the Light into them.

THE ART OF MEDITATION

In approaching the art of meditation, one of the most difficult things is concentration, but here we should use *substitution* rather than *suppression*. We can choose something in which we are really interested, can concentrate on it, and let it lift us to a higher vibration. And we do not all have to meditate in the same way. If we do not allow ourselves to feel inadequate, we shall find hidden capabilities. There may be an incresed efficiency in our daily life simply because we are paying attention, and we shall certainly be greatly enriched. Indeed, even if we do not achieve mystical illumination, it is possible that this new efficiency in daily living may be just as important a step on the path of life.

The soul looks up towards the spirit and receives illumination, and this is then brought down into our everyday lives. We can become like a radio station, tuned in to higher vibrations, and, as we develop, we shall begin to receive impressions, flashes of inspiration from higher sources. This is the development of *intuitional consciousness.* As we progress, we shall become increasingly able to intuit some aspect of the Divine plan, that aspect of it which we personally are led to put into effect. The increasing intuitional consciousness will help us to discover our particular part in the Divine plan. But this will not be achieved by just thirty minutes a day at meditation, helpful as that may be. It requires an hour-by-hour attempt, all day long, to keep our consciousness at the highest possible level, and constant observation to prevent our falling back into a lower vibration. This is our aim, but we must not be alarmed at our failures. We must recognize where we are at the present time.

As William Johnson says, "Finally, it should be remembered that the evolutionary progress is not automatic. It must be carried forward by men and women in ongoing dialogue with one another and with the world." Meditation is a key factor in our evolutionary progress. The meditator or the mystic, going beyond thoughts, images, and concepts to a deeper level of awareness, finds himself in an ever-growing union with the universe and with others, a union which takes place at the core of his being. The mystic is more particularly the builder of the future because he loves. In the last analysis, meditation is a love affair. It is love that builds the earth and carries forward the thrust of evolution.

THE UNCONSCIOUS AND THE SUPERCONSCIOUS

Biofeedback has played quite an important part in teaching people control of the autonomic nervous system and to produce at will the alpha rhythm, the brain rhythm that is most commonly present in meditation. It is tempting to believe that, if we acquire those machines used in biofeedback, we can become splendid meditators. I think it should be emphasized, however, that relaxation and the presence of alpha brain waves are preliminaries to meditation, not meditation itself. A distinction should be drawn between the unconscious and the superconscious. Not all altered states of consciousness are necessarily higher states of consciousness. Drugs can produce expanded awareness, but this is a horizontal, not a vertical, experience. It is interfering with the limiting mechanism of the brain, simply exposing one to other levels of reality, but it is not a spiritual experience. Meditation, however, can put one in touch with higher levels of reality with this intuitive level of consciousness.

Scientists, as we know, are constantly aided in their work by tuning into some higher form of knowledge. They do a great deal of preliminary work and research, and then the flash of inspiration comes when they have switched off, when they are sitting in a bath or climbing on a bus. So one thing that seems absolutely vital to tuning in is this switching-off process, this period of incubation when the seeds are allowed to germinate in darkness. This question of expanded awareness involves developing the intellect and going beyond it to a point where rational thought is put aside. Then, and only then, apparently, can the awareness flow. It is not so much an upward and outward straining; it is seeing what was there all the time. And so it is with meditation. It is not an activity to be strained at, because the whole process of the evolution of consciousness is possible due to the mechanism within us.

While Eastern meditation usually puts rational thought aside, Western meditation frequently adopts a line of rational thought to raise the consciousness, followed by an attempt at listening silence. Either way, the test of meditation is in its practical application in everyday life. Eventually, all types will, I think, be superseded by a continuous soul contact, but not until we have done all the preliminary work. Then every moment of every day will be a meditation.

MEDITATION AS LOVE IN ACTION

In the silence, one can enter into a deeper state of awareness, called in Sanskrit *samadhi*. Sometimes the repetition of a *mantra*, or "sacred words," lift us onto a different level. It may be that repetition switches off rational thought and allows the intuition to flow. I believe that the result of deep meditation is love in action. In

Western mysticism, there is increasingly this form of creative meditation which invokes Light through lifting the consciousness and then pouring it out into the world. Personal development is not an end in itself and is important only as it contributes to a life of service; and service is the means of producing effects on the outward physical plane in a very practical way.

Another great concept is that, through meditation, we can actually participate in the evolution of the planet itself. We know that we ourselves are in the body of this great being, the planet; and humanity, we are told, is the brain tissue of the planetary deity. Each of us has millions of unused brain cells—apparently we use but 10 percent of our brain capacity—and the remainder, at the moment, is undeveloped. We are told that the mass of people are like the millions of unused brain cells; but aspirants, disciples, and those who start to meditate constitute the inner group of vitally alive brain cells. The more powerful their united vibration, the clearer the light which they reflect, the more rapidly will the present inert mass of human cells be brought into activity. So this, too, is a great task, a dramatic task in which we are engaged, our part in the evolution of the planet itself.

We have considered threefold personality as the foundation of the rainbow bridge which first connects the little self to the soul, and then the soul to the spirit. Having developed the intellect, we need to silence it in order to come into this higher form of knowing, which cannot get through when our minds are full of thoughts, or when we are full of tension. In this state, the law of reversed effort takes effect. We need to relax and flow with the forces around us. In the mechanics of meditation, there is, first of all, the act of concentration, when we steadily hold the mind on a chosen word or phrase and we are lifted on to a higher level of awareness. In the next stage, thought is suspended with an attitude of expectancy and of listening. I sometimes think that perhaps this is the difference between prayer and meditation. Prayer, of course, is a very important part of our spiritual lives, but, in meditation, we actually give time to listen to the word of God. Next follows contemplation, when we switch off rational thought and listen. Then, after a time, the soul takes over and itself contemplates. It turns towards the world of the spirit and brings in Light. This is receiving the inspiration of the spirit, to be brought into brain consciousness, and then to be demonstrated in a life of service.

25

Using Herbs Wisely and Effectively

ADELE G. DAWSON

Herbs are safe and easily prepared remedies for many common imbalances which cause annoyance and, sometimes, suffering. One who is ready to take some responsibility for his own health, physical and spiritual, can learn to use herbs for nutritious food and drink, for prevention and cure of disease, and for the joy and peace of regaining attunement with the living earth.

The use of herbs is not new. It dates back 60,000 years to Neanderthal man, whose ritual burials have been found to contain seeds and pollen of medicinal herbs which still grow in the area and are used today for healing.

THE HISTORY OF HERBS

The history of herbs, from the bronze age to the nineteenth century, is also the history of medicine. Fifteen hundred years B.C., the Egyptian Ebers Papyrus listed many of the diseases which plague people today—asthma, colds, colitis, rheumatism, cardiac and skin diseases—as well as herbal formulas for their prevention and cure. Many of the plants recommended in this written herbal can be grown in a small herb garden. Anise, basil, marjoram, dill, coriander, and wormwood all thrive in northern gardens.

Magic and medicine went hand-in-hand in earliest Egypt. But, if we say that magic is an agency that works with wonderful effect, as one dictionary does, this alliance does not seem so strange.

Today, herbal medicine takes its place among the many alternate therapies that holistic health care offers to replace synthetic drugs, which often suppress a symptom without eliminating the cause. There is an ancient precedent for the combined use of herbs and other therapies.

Aesculapius, the legendary physician of ancient Greece, cured patients in Epidaurus, his spa overlooking the Saronic Gulf, by the use of herbs, music, drama, dream interpretation, and serpent worship. The names of some four hundred herbs were engraved on a stone slab which can be seen today in the healing temple at Epidaurus. Invalids came from all parts of Greece to be treated at this first holistic health center. It became the paradigm for all the other healing centers in Greece, presided over by physicians who were called *Aesculapediae.*

THE FOUR CATEGORIES OF HERBS

The use of herbs, past and present, can be divided into four categories: preventive, curative, nutritive, and mood-changing. Many herbs fill an important place in two or more groups. Garlic is an example. In ancient Egypt, it was fed to the workers who built the pyramids; the conquering legions of Rome were given bread with garlic and sesame seeds as their rations when on the march. Modern herbalists use it as a natural antibiotic (it contains sulphur) to prevent and cure colds and sore throat and to heal wounds. Recently, I saw white spots on the skin, due to melanin deficiency, cured by local application of garlic juice.

During the reign of Richard II of England, a salad prepared by the royal chefs contained borage, cresses, fennel, garlic, leeks, mint, onions, purslane, rosemary, and rue. These are herbs which are preventive, curative, mood-changing, and packed with vitamins.

Parsley fits into three slots. It contains minerals and vitamins and is a specific remedy for high blood pressure. Purslane has more vitamin C than even the celebrated rose hip and acerola cherry. It has the added advantage of appearing in everyone's garden, uninvited, and often unappreciated. A low creeping plant with a thick reddish stem and small round succulent leaves, purslane can be used raw in summer salads or cooked as a pot herb. In Mexico, it is sold in the markets, along with cultivated vegetables.

Rosemary and borage, besides their many other virtues, are mood-changing. John Gerard, in his fifteenth-century herbal, said of borage that it was "used everywhere for the comfort of the heart, for the driving away of sorrow, and increasing the joy of the mind." We know that it is also cooling, tonic, and useful in nervous conditions. Small bits of rosemary snipped into a salad can be stimulating and stomachic. Large amounts should not be eaten, as they may prove toxic, but, for external use, an infusion of rosemary is a safe mouthwash. A rinse used after a shampoo prevents the falling of hair. It is a disinfectant for skin wounds, and a cloth dipped in an infusion and placed on the forehead relieves headache.

Watercress and other members of the cress family are diuretic and stimulating, useful in preventing and controlling mucus in the upper respiratory systems.

Both garlic and onions combat infection, prevent putrefaction in the gastro-intestinal tract, and ward off colds and sore throat.

Sage is so well known as a condiment and an herb to enliven the traditional Thanksgiving turkey stuffing that we need only mention a few other virtues. An infusion makes a healing gargle for sore throat and laryngitis. Used as a mouthwash, it tightens up loose teeth. One other specific—it dries up mother's milk when a baby is being weaned.

Rue has a long history in folk medicine as a carminitive (relieves gas pains), as a digestive, and as an emmenagogue (promotes menstruation). It should not be taken in large doses or over a long period of time because it is toxic. Dioscorides, an early Greek herbalist, summed up its virtues and dangers by saying that it was good to cure gout and sciatica and to provoke menstruation, but it should be avoided during pregnancy as it causes abortion. The fact that it was often used as an abortive was thought to be the reason why the late dictator, Francisco Franco, closed the botanical gardens in El Retiro Park in Madrid, which had been founded by order of Charles III circa A.D. 900. Medicinal herbs cultivated there were given free to all who came to seek them. Perhaps the present king will restore the gardens, now in sad condition, and once more make healthful herbs available to the sick and poor.

HERBS IN THE WILD

Many very useful herbs do not need to be cultivated. They are available to us if we walk across an abandoned field or an old logging road, along a brook, or through a wooded area.

Yarrow, tansy, St. Johnswort, agrimony, and evening primrose, all of which thrive in poor, dry soil, can be had for the gathering. Mint and coltsfoot follow clear-running streams, boneset and horsetail like damp locations, while leeks, wild ginger, blue cohosh, and violets are found in the deep humus soil of woodlands.

Every imbalance in the body that causes distress has a remedy in the plant world. Herbal medicine can be learned by anyone; the place to start is where you are. Begin by learning to recognize a few common herbs that grow in your own back yard, on your lawn, or between the cracks in the sidewalk on your street.

Dandelion, plantain, ground ivy, hawkweed, burdock, jewel weed, and the greater celandine are all plants that invade the most urban environment. They are found on small patches of grass near sidewalks and parking lots, around the foundations of buildings, and in the turned soil of the smallest flower beds.

BEGINNING TO USE HERBS

Select an herb that grows near you. Look it up in a wild flower guide, and study its growth habits, leaf and flower arrangement, and color. After you have identified it, look it up by its botanical name in several herb books. Check its medicinal value, the part of the herb which is used, and how to preserve and prepare it. Be sure to check the correct dosage, whether there are any special prohibitions concerning the length of time it may safely be used, and whether it should be used during pregnancy. If it is listed for some common ailment such as bee sting, headache, diarrhea, or hiccoughs, try it the next time you need such a remedy.

After you feel secure in recognizing and using one herb, go on to another. Continue this process until you feel comfortable about using herbs to minister to the needs of your household.

When you begin to use herbs, you may want to start from the other end. Try making a list of the health problems most common in your family. Your list may include colds, sinusitis, indigestion, insomnia, acne. Look in the index of several herb books and read about the herbs recommended for these conditions. If you live in the country, where wild herbs are available, take a walk with a good wildflower guide in hand; use it for identification, and collect what you need. If you are in a town or suburb and have room for a garden, order seeds or get plants from a greenhouse. A third option is buying the dried herbs from a health food store or ordering them from a reliable source of botanicals. In any case, you will find that, in a relatively short time, you will be able to recognize and use the herbs you need to keep your family healthy and happy.

A WORD OF CAUTION

One word of caution: When using herbal remedies, take time to study the cause behind the symptom. If you work only on the symptom, you are falling into the same error that has limited conventional medical care. For example, a headache may be cured by taking an infusion of agrimony, elder flowers, blue vervain, or a number of other herbs. But what is causing the headache? Eyestrain, tension, worry, overexposure to fluorescent light, fatigue, constipation, or a combination of several factors can cause headache. Try to determine and then modify or eliminate the cause as well as the symptom.

THE HERB GARDEN

If you decide to plant an herb garden, start with herbs that can be used as food, drink, condiment, medicine, cosmetic or scent, insect repellent, aesthetic joy, and magic.

Start with squaring the circle. Four tall herbs may be chosen to form corners for a wagon-wheel arrangement of smaller herbs. Comfrey, lovage, wormwood, and sweet cicely are good choices. Comfrey, a handsome plant replete with vitamins and trace minerals, is excellent in salad, as a pot herb, or in a cooling blender drink. Both leaves and root contain alantoin, a cell proliferant which heals both external and internal cuts, bruises, and irritations. The raw green leaves can be used as a bandage on cuts or bruises or as an infusion or poultice. Dried leaves can be made into an infusion which combines well with other herbs that have a stronger flavor, such as mint. This combination as a social tea is healthy, too. A decoction of the comfrey root causes bones to grow together.

Lovage, brought to America by the early English colonists as a celery substitute, is useful as a salad herb when the leaves are young and tender. Later in the summer, they can be dried for winter use in soups and stews. Lovage is mildly stimulating, a diuretic which is useful for urinary problems. An infusion of the leaves used as a wash for the face is popular in Scandinavian countries.

Wormwood tea has long been used as a bitter spring tonic. It will relieve heartburn and gastric discomfort. For centuries, it has been used to get rid of intestinal worms, alone or combined with tansy, garlic, and hyssop. It is also a good insecticide.

Sweet cicely's handsome fernlike leaves and fluffy white blossoms add aesthetic appeal to the garden and are anise-flavored, a pleasant addition to a salad or tea.

All four of these plants are hardy perennials even in very cold winters.

In the small wagon-wheel garden, annual, biannual, and perennial herbs can be arranged according to size and color. Sweet basil and the purple variety called dark opal, marjoram, parsley, anise, chives, fragrant mints, dill, savory, and sweet woodruff are all multi-purpose herbs, culinary and medicinal.

It is interesting to note that, in the oldest description of monastery gardens available, one of St. Gall in Switzerland, we learn that the "physic garden" was placed near the doctor's house. Care of this garden was often a full-time job for a laborer, but the doctor was expected to supervise the work. The garden was divided into eight oblong beds and eight more border plots. Savory, sage, rue, pennyroyal, fenugreek, peppermint, and rosemary were all represented, a good assemblage which we still find useful, fragrant, and aesthetically pleasing today.

The combined effect of scent, color, and the myriad variety of patterns in the herb garden is a built-in therapy. A meditation bench where we can sit, see, and breathe in the purified air from plants with centuries of healing behind them is part of the wise use of herbs.

26

Biofeedback: The Teaching Mirror

ANNE OLIVER BASSAGE

Biofeedback—what is it? It is like a mirror that reflects your deep state of internal health. It teaches you how to be your own healer. It is not a magic instrument that can make you well, but it is a tool that can help you regulate your own psychophysiological states.

FEEDBACK-BIOFEEDBACK

Feedback has been around for a long time. All learning has a feedback component. Looking into a mirror is like biofeedback (feedback from the body); you see a vivid indicator of your physical state; you may see yourself with bloodshot eyes and messy hair, and you say to yourself, "Heavens, I didn't realize I was that bad!" So you take steps to alter the image. The mirror doesn't do it. You brush your hair, abstain from alcohol for a few days, get a little more sleep. You look again and feel satisfaction that you have been able to improve the situation. Biofeedback gets that kind of results and more.

Biofeedback today, while operating on the same principle, includes the use of sophisticated electronic instruments to indicate, to mirror, complex psychophysiological states that we used to think were beyond our reach. Forty-five years ago, at Vassar, I was taught that the autonomic nervous system was just that—automatic—beyond my control; we believed that rate of breathing, blood pressure, sweat, hormone secretions, and all the functions controlled by the sympathetic nervous system could not be regulated by one's will.

204

Barbara Brown, one of the early workers with biofeedback, working at the Sepulveda Veteran's Hospital in California, hit on the principle of biofeedback when she was experimenting with alpha brain waves and light. She was really investigating the problem of communicating about the subjective state. She realized in her experiment that her subject's feelings would be modified by the information he was receiving about his own brain waves. "This was biofeedback," she says.

The use of biofeedback arose simultaneously all over the country; Joseph Kamiya in California, Neal Miller of New York City, Al Ax in Detroit, Joseph Mullholand of New Bedford, Mass., Elmer and Alyce Green in Topeka, Kansas, and many others did pioneer experimental work. Although they were all doing quite different research, they were all using electronic instruments, and they were all heading in the same direction. Biofeedback had to be conceived psychophysiologically, the instrumentation developed, and years of controlled experiments done before it could be used clinically. The idea has spread remarkably quickly because people seem to intuit the truth of the biofeedback experience.

THE ELECTRONIC EXPLOSION

The electronic explosion that came in the period between World War II and the moon shot produced incredibly sensitive transducers, high-gain amplifiers, and complex computer techniques that can convert changes in the autonomic state into meter, light, or sound signals that anyone can understand. Seeing such changes is the first step toward control.

There are many electronic biofeedback instruments used to measure physiological states: the EEG (the electro–encephalograph) that measures brain waves; the GSR (the galvanic skin response instrument) that measures sweat production, usually on the hand; the blood pressure cuff with built-in sound and visual signs. Most of our physiological systems can be measured in some way and instrumented to give biofeedback signals; even the production of acid in the stomach and the secretion of the thyroid gland have been monitored.

The principal instruments now used clinically are the EMG, the electromyograph that measures muscle tension; and the TEMP, an instrument that measures skin temperature. To use the EMG, sensors are placed over the muscle to be tested, and, through these ultrasensitive ears, the tiny electrical firings of muscle fibers are picked up and shown on a meter or by sound from an amplifier. A student can see or hear his muscles contract or relax. Then he notes the inner feeling that occurs when the muscle is deeply relaxed, and, if he wants to bring about that deep relaxation again, he recreates the inner feelings which produce the desired result. Muscle tension is often difficult to feel because we are all used to it; bracing is part of our daily life. After EMG relaxation training, one can recognize tension when it begins and so interrupt a muscle tension buildup.

The temperature instrument shows minute changes in the temperature of the skin by means of a light or dial signal, or it gives a beep that goes up or down in pitch with the rise and fall of the temperature. With the instrument, one can literally see the subjective states as they are going on inside the skin, for the skin is the most sensitive indicator of inner tension. You talk, show emotion, through your fingertips. Seeing the meter rise or fall, a student can learn to control the inner state that is responsible for that change. You see that your hands are warm by watching the meter indicator; you take note of your interior feelings; you increase those feelings and the hand gets warmer and warmer. You are bringing blood down from the head into your arms and hands, and you do it by visualization and imagining inner feelings. A warm hand will abort migraine headaches. We do not know why this happens, but it does.

BIOFEEDBACK RATIONALE

Why is it so important to be able to warm the hands? Hand temperature is almost entirely dependent on blood flow. Blood flow is determined by the diameter of small arteries, and this diameter is determined by smooth muscles that are controlled by the sympathetic nervous system. It follows that if the hand temperature can be regulated, then the sympathetic nervous system has been brought under control. So, warmth in the hands is an indicator of deep autonomic relaxation.

All biofeedback training is based on the psychophysiological principle that says that every change in the physiological state is followed by a change in the mental–emotional state, conscious or unconscious; and, to an equal extent, every change in the mental-emotional state is followed by an appropriate change in the psychophysiological state.

How can this be used by a student to promote health? The answer lies in a combination of self-suggestion and visualization.

Autogenic phrases (phrases which arise from the self, self-suggestion) are used to help the student relax. He is asked to repeat quietly to himself the phrases the teacher gives him—phrases suggesting comfort, heaviness, warmth. This brings about a state of deep relaxation which the therapist recognizes by reading the instruments.

The student is now instructed to use visualization: "Visualize; imagine what you want your body to do; tell your hand to warm, then relax and let the body take over." This is acting on the principle set forth above. A mental-emotional state is created, which in turn creates the physiological state called for. This is control.

When this kind of internal control is learned, it is not lost. It is like learning to ride a bike; once the technique is learned, it is never forgotten. Therefore, one of the goals of biofeedback training is to wean a student away from the instruments. The more quickly this can be achieved, the more the teacher can feel that learning has been successful.

BIOFEEDBACK AND STRESS

Today, biofeedback essentially teaches the control of stress. Hans Selye, the great Montreal authority on stress, says it is not stress that kills us but the way one's body reacts to stress. Some stress is beneficial, and the body must have it; we could not walk or run without stress, and many of the joys in life are achieved by overcoming stress. But bad stress—distress—can kill us.

Take, for example, my high blood pressure. My doctor told me I must relax and slow down, and I tried to let go, to take it easy, but I was not successful. The very knowledge of the necessity for relaxation made me anxious and drove my blood pressure up instead of down. Then my body became used to this higher pressure and the higher pressure became normal for me. Under more daily stress (and we all have it continuously), the cycle began all over again and the pressure mounted still higher. Now even a slight crisis could send the pressure too high, and I would risk the inevitable crippling stroke like the one that ended my mother's life.

Today, the more we learn about various illnesses and metabolic disorders, the more we find that stress is one of the causes of that kind of dis-ease. Stress is well known as a major cause of high blood pressure, ulcer, colitis, headaches, Raynaud's disease, and asthma, and it is also a factor in depression, anxiety, phobias, alcoholism, insomnia, heart problems, learning disabilities, social anxieties (like unemployment) and even cancer.

In biofeedback, we use both the EMG and the TEMP instruments along with relaxation exercises, autogenic phrases, and the use of visualization. This combination gives the student control of subtle processes which had been only in his unconscious and which had therefore been outside his control. The training brings the unconscious to the conscious mind. It makes the student the instrument of his own healing. It reduces stress.

A TEMP TRAINING SESSION

When I begin work with a biofeedback student, I spend the first hour discussing the rationale behind the instrumentation. I use a diagram developed by Elmer and Alyce Green of the Menninger Foundation to explain self-regulation of the psychophysiological events in the conscious and unconscious mind. I also discuss visualization and autonomic phrases, and I answer any questions that arise. Then we talk over that student's particular needs and why he came for biofeedback training, and we set the goals for the entire program.

While attaching the TEMP instrument to the student, I explain what the instrument does and how to read the signals. At the end of a long wire is a small thermistor, like the bulb of a thermometer, which I tape to the middle finger of the dominant hand. The student now makes himself comfortable on a bed or in a reclining chair, closes his eyes, and we begin the relaxing process with autogenic phrases suggesting quietness, heaviness, warmth, and relaxation. The student repeats each phrase quietly to himself after me, and I record on a phrase sheet the temperature changes that show deviation from the starting temperature. Hand temperature may vary from 60 to 95 degrees in a normal person, and this is independent of the temperature of the room. The starting temperature is read from a digital-dial potentiometer which is used to zero the needle on the dial at starting time. The needle shows an increase in temperature when it moves to the right and a decrease when it moves to the left.

When the autonomic phrases have been completed, the student has achieved deep relaxation. His attention is brought back to the room, and he is asked to write a few sentences about his body feelings, thoughts, or emotions during the session. Then we discuss those reactions and correlate them with actual temperature changes as shown on the chart.

Before the end of the session, the student, with eyes open, watches the dial as he repeats the phrases to himself. He can see the needle move to the right if he reacts well to the self–suggestions. This feedback reinforces his ability to relax, to let go, and he will relax further. Seeing the needle act as he wills it to, the student examines how he feels inside. His hands may feel a bit swollen, or have a tingling sensation, or he may feel blood flowing down his arm. He now knows that when he reproduces this inner feeling his hand will warm.

If, however, he approaches his own work with the TEMP saying, "I can never do it," the dial probably will show a decrease in temperature.

I then intervene and say, "You see, you really have fine control. The instrument is doing exactly as you said it would."

He tries harder, and the temperature continues to drop. It drops quickly one degree, two, three and a half. In exasperation the student says, "I give up. I simply can't make it work, no matter how hard I try."

I engage his attention for a few moments by discussing his frustration, and while he is not watching the dial, the hand temperature rises. I ask him to look at the meter, and he will be surprised to see the increase.

"But I didn't do anything," he says.

"You did," I answer, "you learned the second lesson: not to try too hard."

What we need is a passive volition. A paradox? Perhaps, but you must tell the body, "Hands warm," then turn your attention away from the hands and concentrate on comfortable inner relaxation. The body has its own well–being, and, if instructed and left alone, will return to its healthy state. In trying to get to sleep, one sometimes finds that sleep is elusive. If we say, "I'm going to sleep. I'm going to sleep. I'm going to sleep," it just won't work. We're trying too hard. If, instead, we think of a favorite place, imagine it as vividly as possible, recreate the sights, the smells, the sounds, the feelings, the ambience, then we drift off to sleep.

It is the same with biofeedback training; no matter which instrument you are working with, a passive volition is necessary. This skill is sometimes hard to explain to a student and it takes a bit of learning. But seeing the movement of the TEMP meter needle and equating that movement with an inner state is the first step toward control. Inner sensations are brought to consciousness, and the student realizes that to get the results he wants he must reproduce those feelings. I have never had a student who could not learn this.

At the end of the first session, I ask the student to practice the autogenic phrases and relaxation twice a day at home and keep notes of each practice session. The practice sessions are important, as is the note taking. The student and I must be able to evaluate the home sessions; writing about them makes the student think about each practice and jells the experience for him.

In subsequent sessions, I introduce the student to electromyograph (EMG) relaxation, using Edmund Jacobsen's Progressive Relaxation technique, which is essentially relaxation of all the muscles of the body starting with the hand and ending with the toes. Visualization of the process is also an important part of this training. I ask the student to see each muscle, imagine it, understand its use and feel its complete relaxation.

As training develops, I ask the student to replace the autogenic phrases with his own visualization. He may imagine his hand on the hot deck of a sailboat with the sun warming the wood and his hand. As he becomes more adept at hand warming, he may not need the visualizations but may be able to replace these instructions to his body with a kinetic, subjective feeling which is impossible to describe.

Deep breathing is also part of the instruction, diaphragmatic breathing without pauses at intake or expulsion of breath. Breathing, used many times a day for quick relaxation, helps the student incorporate the practice of relaxation into his life. I ask the student to do deep breathing at the times of those small repetitious events that happen every day. If the telephone rings, take several deep breaths before you answer. At a red light, don't fret because you've been delayed, but think, "This is an opportunity to do my deep breathing," take three or four deep breaths, and the red light will seem to turn to green more quickly.

AN INDIVIDUAL PROCESS

The number of sessions is usually set by the student. I ask beginning students to come twice a week at first, but sessions can come further apart as they progress. It is hard to know how many sessions will be useful because each person's needs are different, and each student's response to the teaching varies. Biofeedback is a very private and individual process. One cannot compare one student's progress with another's because a student's genetic inheritance is distinct, his state of health is particular, his will to learn is his own, and his response to subjective feelings is unique.

In all this training, if a student is on medication of any kind, I consult with his physician. This is necessary because the relaxation training often quickly decreases the need for medication, and taking the prescribed amount of the drug could become dangerous. For example, after relaxation training, blood pressure medication might relax the arteries so much that a patient's pressure could fall too low. This must be guarded against. Even if he is not taking a medication, I like to consult with a student's physician. Many doctors do not know about biofeedback, and explaining the results is the best way to introduce them to this fine therapeutic tool.

RESULTS OF TRAINING

After the third or fourth session, many of my students report, "My family says I'm easier to get along with," or "I had the best talk with my husband I've had in ages." This is because the relaxation training improves a student's self-image. If he is learning to control unconscious processes, he is learning self-regulation, and this is a positive reinforcement for a better idea of himself. Somehow the critical, judgmental, argumentative faculties are reduced, and a student will let his true self shine forth. We all have potential that we keep covered. This cover-up is a defense, just as any psychosomatic illness is a defense. Most of us are as sensitive as a sea anemone and have learned to hide that vulnerability by one defense or another. But a stronger self–image removes the necessity for defenses, and healing begins when one gradually lets go.

Another unexpected side effect is the loss of the desire to smoke or drink. Many say, "I noticed that I just don't need cigarettes so much," or "I only take one drink before dinner now. I haven't tried to cut down. I just don't want a second drink as I used to."

The first benefit I noticed from my own biofeedback training was an ability to sleep better. I could drop to sleep quickly, and if I woke during the night, I could sleep again without a long period of thoughts and fantasies accompanied by much turning and adjusting of pillows.

My own psychic powers were released by my biofeedback training. From childhood, I had realized that I had another way of knowing. In college, I learned to call it psychic and to distrust it profoundly. It wasn't scientific, and, above all things, I was a scientist. Now I have learned to trust my hunches, and my life has been enhanced. The Buddhists ask a student to disregard psychic happenings, saying they are distracting and divert one from the Path. I have found them amusing and useful; I no longer deny them.

To me, the most serendipitous gift of biofeedback relaxation training has been the amount of energy it gave me—physical, sexual, creative energy. It was incredible to me. I was sixty-two years old, yet I felt surges of strength race through my body, such strength as I had not felt since I was in college. The waves of energy came at odd unexpected moments—lying in bed, sitting at a concert, cooking dinner. They made me more productive. I could do more more efficiently. I was more centered. I had greater staying power.

Where does the energy come from? A rational explanation would be that the physical energy used in bracing, in both physical and mental defense positions, is made available by deep relaxation. Energy is no longer taken up with useless muscle contractions and so is released for a more constructive life.

Both the Yogis and the Buddhists have a different explanation. They name the power *kundalini,* or coiled energy, and direct it toward certain *chakras* (etheric organs of the body) which are sensitive to superconscious states of being. They say this energy lies latent in the lumbar–spinal region of a human being and operates only partially in educated people, but in those who have learned to induce *samadhi*,* it operates fully. Many Yogis and Buddhists devote their lives to learning self-regulation, and, after years of practice, can control the autonomic nervous system to an astonishing degree. Swami Rama, from Rishekish, India, submitted to the most rigorous scientific testing in the research facilities of the Menninger Foundation. Dr. Elmer and Alyce Green report that the Swami could demonstrate the control of blood vessels in his right hand by choosing two locations two inches apart and in two minutes create a temperature difference of ten degrees in those two spots. He also stopped his heart from pumping blood for seventeen seconds without any indication of tension on the EMG. This was easier to do, he said, than temperature control. Such men can teach us a great deal about awareness and control, yet for years we have ignored their skills and said their claims were somehow faked. Today, medical science is beginning to realize that the teachings of the Eastern mystics can give valuable clues to the nature of consciousness and the function of volition in our lives.

POTENTIAL OF AUTONOMIC CONTROL

Autogenic training was developed in Germany in the early 1900's by Johannes Schultz and today is continued by his pupil, Dr. Wolfgang Luthe. In Vienna, Freud had brought about some remarkable cures of mental illness by his use of hypnosis. One of the reasons he discontinued hypnosis was that it was not suitable for all his patients; some of them resisted. Schultz reasoned that if a patient were to hypnotize himself, this would eliminate resistance. So he developed what he called autogenic (arising from the self) training. Biofeedback can speed up the autogenic training in a remarkable way because, with the instruments, the student actually sees or hears what is happening inside his body. He does not have to rely on a description of a subjective state by his teacher, nor on trial and error practices. Scientific instruments actually measure psychophysiological responses, and seeing these measurements is the first step in control.

---

* *Samadhi:* a state in which the mind is cleared of thought waves and is capable of super-conscious awareness, in which it achieves identity or sameness with the object of concentration.

Deep autonomic relaxation produces two interesting kinds of therapeutic results. When the body has become deeply relaxed, it can often reveal diagnostic information. The relaxation of the autonomic system creates a hypnogogic state of consciousness, the state between waking and sleeping that is not dreaming, though it is like dreaming. It is rather an inward-turned alertness in which the mind is very much in tune with the body. In this state, imagery occurs; vivid auditory, visual, kinesthetic images seem to pop into consciousness without the student's will. These images are as real as dreams or more real, and yet the student is aware that they are not dreams. The images often tell the student the cause of his basic physical problem. Schultz called this "getting answers from the unconscious."

The second possibility which occurs when deep autonomic relaxation takes place is programming of the mind. The body organs and systems, as well as emotions, psychological problems, and obsessive thoughts, can be modified in accordance with the student's desires. This modification might be called self-hypnosis, but whether it is called self–hypnosis or autogenic training or self-suggestion, it works. The same results can be achieved through meditation, autogenic training alone, or other methods, but biofeedback relaxation training with visualization speeds up the autonomic process. Someone has even called it instant Yoga!

BIOFEEDBACK IN THE FUTURE

A real understanding of the tremendous power of biofeedback training creates visions of a future society of self–regulated individuals who could have significant influence in the control of the myriad problems facing us today, some of which threaten our very existence.

But, being more immediately practical, imagine the effect of biofeedback training in our schools. If, by biofeedback training, a six–year–old were taught how to control test anxiety, to diminish his aggressive tendencies, to center his learning ability, to increase his memory, to regulate his own mental health, to remove the threat of mental illness, to let hypnogogic fantasies help him develop his creative powers, to grasp transpersonal values, what a change in education we would see! There is already evidence of a trend toward a more humanistic approach to education, with more emphasis on self–awareness, self–regulation, and holistic health.

However, biofeedback as a tool to study consciousness most engages my speculation. What is man? Who am I? This question, which has haunted man since he became self-conscious, still remains unanswered. If we add the new science of psychophysics to the study of consciousness, we then explore a dimension which has been lost to us since the time of Descartes, namely the interacting effects of the body and the mind. We are learning that mind is a force in nature both inside the skin and outside, and that is as mind-shaking a concept as the change in thought brought about by Einstein.

We are once again on the threshold of a New Age.

27

The Wholing Process: Conscious Self-Healing

LOUISE SUNFEATHER

Contemporary science has taught us much about the nature of the universe. Sub-atomic physics shows that reality consists of two simultaneous phenomena, particles and waves; that everything is energy in motion, vibrating between two poles; that *matter* is energy manifest as form; that energy is neither created nor destroyed but merely changes form; that the act of observation affects and is affected by the phenomenon being observed; that every individual expression of energy is part of a larger complex pattern of energy at the same time.

These are important concepts in the understanding of human evolution, which is that movement from the part to the whole, from our separate, limited existences back to our source, the limitless All. That movement, as we claim both our "particlehood" (our individualness, our self) and our "waveness" (our collectiveness, our Divine Self), is also the path of healing, or *wholing*. We see that we, all of who we are, are manifestations in physical form of energy in motion, energy moving between two poles, vibrating in harmony and balance or out of harmony. We see that the act of observation, the being aware, the identification of our consciousness with an event or thought, has some relationship with that form. We see we can use our acts of observation to help energy change form, to unblock the obstructions, to free the flow. We see that we are evolving beings, who are and who can be actively responsible for our own evolution. For our own self-healing. For our wholing.

216

WHAT WHOLING MEANS

Wholing refers specifically to the reclaiming or remembering of lost or undiscovered fragments of the self, bringing the pieces into harmonious relationship with each other and with the larger Divine Self. Clearly, if we identify our consciousness with ourselves as fragments, as separate from all other existence, and from our own source of wholeness, we restrict the flow of energy or life force and create blocks to our vitality. In many cases, these blocks manifest as dis-ease or imbalance. If, on the other hand, we identify our consciousness with wholeness, with the interconnectedness of all existence, we have available to us all that we need to be whole and in harmonious relationship with ourselves, others, and our environment. The *wholing process*, then, refers to the ongoing process by which we learn to identify our consciousness with our wholeness and our oneness with the life force, and to accept and appreciate our "all-here-ness."

We all grew up in a world founded on the premise of reductionism, which seeks to reduce the universe to its component parts. For all of us, then, the full identification with wholeness requires a shift in world view or basic premise, a relearning of the true nature of the universe, which is the interrelatedness of all parts forming a whole which is greater than the sum of its parts. Since our world view determines what we see and how we act, we lay down patterns of responses which, over time, become fixed and familiar, and often far removed in conscious awareness from the original world view or focus of consciousness that created them. Our work, then, is to discover those patterns which express a sense of limitation or separation; to see them and their effects clearly, to bring them into the light of our consciousness, and, by doing so, transform them into new patterns which express our new world view of wholism.

AREAS OF RELATIONSHIP

The five basic areas of relationship in which our world views determine how we live are:

1. the relationship of the self with the self;

2. the relationship of the self with others;
3. the relationship of the self with the planet, or natural world;
4. the relationship of the self with the cosmos;
5. the relationship of the self with its own evolution.

Let us examine each of these areas in turn, seeking to understand how our basic world view determines the patterns of our lives and is, therefore, available as raw material to be transformed.

Relationship of Self to Self

This is the realm of self-definition or self-image. We come to believe certain things about our bodies, our minds, our feelings, our higher nature, based on what we hear and observe from the significant others in our lives. Children, by their physical nature dependent on others for their survival, interpret the data from their environment in terms of "Who and how must I be in order to survive in this world—i.e., to get what I need emotionally, physically, etc.?" Conforming to family and culture norms almost always means shutting off parts of ourselves. Most of us grow up with the shoulds and shouldn'ts of our significant others reflected in our self-image and consequently in our relationships with all others. These limitations are fully registered as well in the structure and development of our physical bodies. The basic questions, "Am I entitled to be myself, all of who I am? Am I entitled to be alive, to be all here?" become keys to a true sense of the whole self.

Relationship of Self to Others

This is the area of human economics, and involves issues of how we give and receive that which we need for human intercourse in groups of any size and any degree of intimacy. All relationships involve two simultaneous forces, attraction and repulsion. In human groups, these forces are experienced as differentiation and fusion, or autonomy and interdependence, centripetal and centrifugal energy. "How do I maintain my uniqueness and still be part of the larger entity called 'us'?" is the basic struggle of all interpersonal relationships. From our families and communities we learn personal patterns of response to the tension created by these simultaneous forces, and eventually we become locked into behavioral habits that act out our assumptions about relationships. A reductionist culture teaches us to withold our resources and try to manipulate others to get some of theirs, and to foster dependency (I need you) or counterdependency (I don't need anyone. I can do it all myself.). How to live interdependently, recognizing and utilizing the gifts of all, is our work in this area.

Relationship of Self with the Planet

This is the realm of economics of natural resources, and affects how we give to and take from the earth itself and all other forms of creation. Again, as children, we learn from what we see around us how and what our connection is with our larger physical ecosystem; here, too, we develop assumptions and basic views on what is real and correct. What we come to believe about "man" and "nature" determines how we treat and experience the natural forces. Are we victors and victims, or are we co-creators? Do we seek to own or take from nature for our own gain, or do we recognize our mutuality and interrelatedness? Do we build strip mines or sundance arbors? Slaughter whales or learn from their singing?

Relationship of Self to Cosmos

This is the metaphysical area, and provides the spiritual and moral structure by which we live as individuals and as groups. "Who or what is God?" is the ultimate question here. Is there some higher force and does it reside in a great being "out there," or is it somehow inside each self? What is good and what is evil, and how can we live correctly? How are the mysteries of the universe related to our lives? Are we apart from them or a part of them? Alone or all one?

Relationship of Self with Its Own Evolution

Given that all energy is in motion, that change is the nature of our lives, we are all in a continual process of change and development. To observe that process, to participate in it, extracting the lessons and the essence of our experiences, letting go of old forms that no longer work and risking new patterns, to consciously direct through our will that journey toward wholeness, is to acknowledge our relatedness with the universe. Imagining that we are victims or pawns of evolution (I can't help it; it all happens *to* me!) or denying the potential of change (That's just the way I am/things are.) are expressions of our separateness.

When we identify in ourselves, as we all do, patterns in any of these five areas based on assumptions of separateness, the process of wholing is the process of transforming the old pattern into a new one. How does that happen?

The alchemical process of turning dross to gold provides a clear picture of the process of transformation. The steps are basically to dissolve or discharge the old material and resolve or recharge the new. The first step is awareness.

FIRST STEP TOWARD CHANGE

When we see clearly just where we are, and where a particular block or resistance to the free flow of energy has come from in our history, we have already taken the first major step toward changing it. This is what is meant by bringing something into the light of consciousness. Awareness can move no further, however, if there is judgment attached to it. If, for instance, we see that we have blocked ourselves from expressing our feelings all our lives because we wanted to please our parents, who insisted we "be good," that block is not free to be transformed if we then invest our energy in being angry with ourselves for having held back or in being angry with our parents for "what they did to us." When we can detach ourselves from any judgment and simply accept what *is*, then we are ready to take the next step in transformation, which is to see what *could be*. When we identify our consciousness with our ideal or vision, we are withdrawing the energy that had been tied up supporting the old pattern, thus discharging or dissolving that pattern and redirecting energy to support a new way of being that expresses our wholeness. We are then able to act differently.

Sometimes, however, we are so strongly identified with our sense of limitation that it is not so simple to withdraw our energy and redirect our consciousness. Often we have to fully confront the block (or pain, or symptom, or dis-ease) as a monster of our own creation, move into it to discover its life-affirming essence or gift. If we recognize that every blockage or pain represents a holding on or resistance to being fully here, and if we know that this blockage contains a lesson available to us, we are then able to extract the essence and let go of the form. Then we can rebuild a new form that supports the quality or ideal we now wish to express.

Considering the wholing process in terms of physical illness and its relationship to our basic world views and attitudes, let us look at some examples of how this understanding of the process of transformation can directly affect our wholing.

We have said that our attitudes or world view provides the basis of how our consciousness gets directed in our lives, and that, further, our bodies directly express that consciousness. Thus, for most people, the basic work of wholing is about claiming the right to be alive and the will to be fully here. Discovering the germ or seed thought that originated the closing off of the life flow in a particular area, and transforming it into a new seed thought of wholeness or completeness can be a dramatic and effective way to work. This work can be done by using the medium of sound, the power of the creative work, to express what is and affirm what could be.

The first step is awareness, discovering the underlying (and often unconscious) statement of which a physical or emotional pain is an expression. For instance, one woman I worked with was not allowed to express any anger as a child. Her basic statement was, "I have to be a good little girl." She had channeled the blocked anger into fits, actually fits of rage, that took the form of epileptic seizures. Another woman was seriously overprotected in her family and believed she could not support herself. She developed mysterious weakness in her legs. Another woman, who experienced being abandoned frequently as a child, decided she would never get close to anyone, including herself. She fabricated, quite literally, a brain tumor that was to make sure she got "cut off."

Seeing and experiencing directly the correlation between the original thought and physical symptom can be relatively simple. The epileptic woman was simply asked what she did with her anger all those years. Where in her body did she put it? The woman with the brain tumor, when asked to show what it meant to be cut off from herself and others, collapsed to the ground, covered her head, and reported feeling dead.

CREATING A NEW PATTERN

The next step, of seeing what could be and transferring the energy into the new pattern of consciousness, can also be done with statements. People can come up with new statements that reflect the opposite of what they have been believing, or what they would like to believe. This usually gets right at the assertion of wholeness. For the woman with epilepsy, the statement became, "I'm entitled to have all my feelings." For the woman with weak legs, the positive statement was, "I can stand on my own two feet." For the woman with supposed brain cancer, it became, "I can be in contact with myself; I'm entitled to be alive!"

Simply making the positive statement is a powerful experience, but not the end of the process. The new view must be integrated into the whole being, allowing for the discharge of the energy stored in the old pattern and concretizing the restructured vision. The block created by the original attitude can be directly addressed and released. This could happen in any number of ways: though visualization, movement, body work, drawing, chanting, etc. To continue with' the use of the positive seed-statement, the next step would be for the person to make his new statement from deep inside. If in a group setting, the person can go around the circle, making eye contact with each person and saying the new statement. If other people are not present, trees, plants, imaginary people, or even pillows will do. In the process of repeating from deep within the new positive attitude, the person inevitably comes directly into contact with the block of energy that the old one had engendered.

DISCHARGING AND RECHARGING

Each repetition of the affirmation brings an increasingly direct confrontation between the old and the new pattern, and, if the person is ready to accept the restructuring, this confrontation will create a discharge as the old gives way to the new statement of will. Discharge comes in many forms, the most common being crying, laughing, shaking, blowing, trembling, or even vomiting. The discharge is not an end in itself, being merely the release of waste energy, and the person should be encouraged to continue the affirmation process right through whatever discharge is occurring. This then becomes the recharge stage, where consciousness is shifted and identification occurs with wholeness and expression of the life force rather than separateness and a closing off or repressing of part of the whole.

The recharge is the proper place for encouragement. The new attitude, overcoming as it does a powerful and time-honored blockage, needs to be set and integrated throughout the whole person. This can be done from the inside through meditation, prayer, or visualization, and can be helped from the outside by offering encouragement, appreciation, or physical or verbal "strokes." Once the person has acknowledged that he can take responsibility for his own wholing through identifying his consciousness with positive patterns and expressions of wholeness, then other resources to help that happen are most effective—herbs, diet, massage, friendships, music, all the so-called wholistic approaches. These and many other healing resources help the individual fully integrate the new world views or expressions of life-consciousness, as the process is a continuing one of awareness, discharge, and recharge; of seeing how we have identified our consciousness with limitation, letting go, reidentifying with wholeness, and moving as if it were so.

Once the process has started by the initial act of will, the organism will naturally throw into consciousness those areas which it is ready to transmute. The self can always know where the next step is, the next place to discharge and recharge, by experiencing where the pain is, pain being the resistance to letting go. Moving into the pain or energy block, discovering through asking the right questions what that block is an expression of, becomes itself the new behavior rather than shrinking from the pain or assuming one has no control over it.

A CHAIN OF REACTIONS

Because body, mind, and spirit are all aspects of one entity, and because all five areas of relationship mentioned earlier are interrelated, as consciousness changes in one area it affects others. Thus, an initial act of aligning the will with the desire to be all here, fully alive, may produce a whole chain of reactions, as the restructuring radiates from the seed or core outward, affecting ever more aspects of the self. The more we contact and integrate the different aspects of our self, the more we move into our true Self, or Divine Wholeness. That journey or wholing process is available to anyone ready to let go of the fear and resistance to being fully alive and to claim active participation in his own wholing. It is a journey we share in common and can help each other with.

It is a journey many of us can no longer afford to hesitate about. Our planet is at an evolutionary critical-choice point. We can destroy ourselves through war, hatred, separation, and abuse of human and physical resources, or re-create ourselves and our human structures from the inside out, healing the vast wounds that have already been sustained. The choice is whether or not to commit our will and resources to wholeness and planetary healing, and to take responsibility for that process. Our individual wholing is an essential ingredient to the larger planetary process; the same choices, commitment, and transformations are involved regardless of the level of organization. We can no longer afford to sit and wait for it to happen "to" us. We can claim our right to be whole and alive and acknowledge our power to heal ourselves, individually and collectively. We can claim all of who we are. We can be the particle and the wave. We can be whole.

28

Foot Reflexology and Prenatal Therapy

BARBARA D'ARCY-THOMPSON

The pressure of the hands causes the springs of
life to flow
TOKUJIRO NANIKOSHI

W|hat is the essence of healing? Is there a quality, a
talent, that enables some people to be healers,
which others of us lack? No, we are all healers. In
our every word and action and movement, and, above all, in the
touch of our hands, we are healers. Foot reflexology is a method of
maintaining health of body that was known thousands of years
ago by the Chinese, Japanese, and Indonesians. Aware that the
health of the body and the health of the feet are interdependent,
they made the discovery that every organ, every area in the entire
body, has a corresponding reflex point in other parts of the body;
the most sensitive are those on the feet, with secondary points on
the hands and the head. These reflexes are fifteen to twenty times
as sensitive as the organs themselves, and, unlike them, are accessible and easily stimulated. The practitioner, his fingers working
with deep compression massage on the reflex areas, discovers and
relieves disharmony or imbalance in the corresponding organs.

DR. WILLIAM FITZGERALD AND ZONE THERAPY

In the early years of this century, an American doctor, William H.
Fitzgerald, M.D., made a study of the ancient Chinese systems of
healing. He recognized that the human body functions in accordance with the laws of polarity, the head and the feet being the
poles between which pass pathways, channels or currents of en-

ergy, whose circulation is essential to keep the body in balance and vitality. There is a strong link here with acupuncture and other ancient allied therapies.

Dr. Fitzgerald divided the body longitudinally into ten zones, each one starting in the head and passing down through the body to end in the tips of the toes, inclusive of all organs in its path; the zones going through the shoulders and arms end in the tips of the fingers and thumbs.

The brain, sinuses, eyes, and ears have their reflexes in the toes; continuing down through the foot are the reflexes of the thyroid, the lungs, and the internal organs; around the heels and the Achilles tendon are the organs of reproduction and elimination. The upper surfaces of the feet reflect the framework, the soles the internal organs. The reflexes of the spine lie on the inner side of both feet from the first joint of the big toe along the bony arch to below the ankle bone, ending at the top of the heel bone.

HEALING ON MANY LEVELS

In foot reflexology, we are healing on many levels. As the work begins, we dedicate ourselves to the highest good of the patient; there is an outflowing of energy, caring, and love that pours through us and through the tips of our fingers. Before actually touching the patient's feet, one moves slowly and gradually through his "energy field" until it feels right to establish contact.

Then follows a gentle all-over massage of the feet and legs, working from the toes toward the ankles, and upward to the knees; the hands move where it feels right for them to be. Through the nerve endings in the feet, we are soothing and relaxing the whole system, and, through pressure on the capillaries, the circulatory system is stimulated; meanwhile, blockages in the energy channels are removed. Working all over the foot with pressure of the fingers and thumbs, one finds points or areas of sensitivity or pain. One watches the patient's face for his reactions and asks for "feedback." Painful areas are treated with great care, the pain being "evened out" so that it is not too drastic. Usually, the patient will tell you that, although it really hurts, it is a "good pain"; in other words, he feels it is doing good, and he is prepared to put up with it.

It sometimes happens that, at a first treatment, a patient's feet register no sensations. They are, as it were, just blocks, and insensitive; in subsequent treatments, they "come alive." Occasionally, as in other natural therapies, a person in poor health may feel not better but worse after the first treatment; the dis-eased pattern of his body is having to change, and toxins are being released into his system. As the new pattern becomes established, he feels a different person.

When circulation has become congested and energy channels blocked, waste materials in the form of tiny acid crystals are deposited, through gravity, on the nerve endings of the feet. As they are rubbed out between the fingers and thumb, the patient can feel a jab of acute pain, but afterwards he will tell you that he is "walking on air." Reflexology helps not only the organs of the body, but all their attendant functions as well, thus attaining balance.

REFLEXOLOGY AS A MEANS OF DIAGNOSIS

As a means of diagnosis, reflexology is readily applied and wonderfully accurate; it can give warning of troubles long before they become apparent. All physical conditions respond to treatment, but, especially, the whole system is relaxed. As you practice reflexology, you never cease to wonder at this remarkable therapy, and are amazed at the ever-expanding revelation of the marvels of the human body.

ROBERT ST. JOHN'S DISCOVERY

From reflexology came a development of the utmost importance. Robert St. John, a man with an inquiring, rational mind who was also a highly intuitive person, had been a practitioner in England for a number of years; but always, at the back of his mind, he felt there was something more to this therapy, something of great importance, that had not yet been discovered. One day, in an intuitive flash, it came to him that there is one other quite astonishing reflex in the feet. This reflex belongs to the prenatal period, the nine-month gestation period in the womb. It is something intangible, belonging to the past, but nevertheless it has its own reflex area, and, as we work on it, we are evoking the characteristics that were laid down in the past.

We are not, however, looking at the past as something gone forever. Time is more like a river that flows from a lake into the sea, whence moisture is taken up into the atmosphere to return again to the earth and repeat the cycle. The events of the past are still in some form of existence, and, as we bring them back into focus, we can release them from the hold of time. As reflexology releases stresses and blocks in the organs of the body, this therapy releases patterns of stress and blocks that were set up "in time," in the thirty-eight weeks of the gestation period.

The reflex area is that of the spine. Dr. Frederick Leboyer, in his book *Birth Without Violence*, shows how the spine, being so closely linked to the central nervous system, holds every memory of all our life; memories since our birth and before it, memories that go back to the beginning of time; every terror, every anguish associated with birth as we in the West are accustomed to it, is recorded in the spine and its reflexes, and there, unless released, they remain.

Prenatal Therapy

St. John called his work *prenatal therapy*, unfortunately a confusing term. It has not, as the words suggest, anything to do with expectant mothers, but is concerned with the prenatal reflexes. He also uses the term *metamorphosis*, since the treatment enables people to undergo radical changes. The clarity of motivation in the practitioner is an important factor in the treatment. Prenatal therapy differs from most other therapies in which the medical profession gives help to the patient from outside of himself; in such cases, the pattern of change may or may not be permanent. In prenatal therapy, we are concerned with the person only, not with his symptoms or illness. We must be centered in ourselves, clear and detached in our minds, so that we may induce these qualities in the mind of the patient. We are simply catalysts, concerned only for awakening in the patient his own inner sense of action. He will initiate the changes he knows to be necessary; the movement is from within, from the center outwards. His own vital energy, his will to live, his passion for life, all that is entailed in being human, will work to bring about the changes that will restore him to normality and wholeness.

The work itself is very simple. It consists of massage and manipulation of the spinal reflexes on both feet, which, as we saw in our earlier talk about reflexology, lie from the big toe through the arch of the foot to the heel.

Prenatal Therapy and the Retarded Child

As the pattern of his new work was beginning to unfold, St. John had occasion to treat a mongoloid child a few weeks old. After a year of treatment, such transformation had taken place that she was in every way a completely normal child. This experience so impressed him that he determined to devote a considerable part of his time to working with mentally handicapped children. He came to realize that it is possible to restore such children to complete normality of mind and body, provided they are still young enough not to have established too rigid a mental and physical pattern.

> Even the worst of retarded conditions is changeable, whether the child be mongoloid, spastic, autistic or paralysed, the inner ability to change applies to every case; change is possible from within the child, and by his own ability he can re-create his primary structure. . . . I have become aware that under the surface of their inability to express and to function normally, there is a very normal mind, consciously thinking normally and wishing to express itself normally as others do. . . . The average retarded child is hiding behind a block of fear, resistance and tension. Treatment has the effect of starting an action which is the child's own way of dealing with the problem that his life presents to him.

The limiting factors would be an environment in which there is lack of care, real lack of understanding of the changes the child will undergo, and extreme defectiveness, where a child is sunk so far into abnormality that he has never been able to make contact with life at all.

St. John divides the gestation period into five stages, preconception, conception, postconception, prebirth and birth. At each of these stages, the characteristics of the developing consciousness, both positive and negative, mental and physical, are laid down, and it is here that originate patterns of stress which will have permanent effects on the nature of the child.

Before conception, the consciousness is approaching the single cell of its new life; this period embraces the whole of history from the beginning of time, all human, all racial, all family inheritance, the relationship of parents, whether or not the child was wanted, and many other factors. If these inherited traits and environmental influences are against normality, there is a reluctance to enter life. This blocking of the spontaneous action of the consciousness produces the inhibited and retarded child.

The second stage, conception, is the first real challenge to the consciousness. It is the entry into matter, which is also the beginning of the time factor of life. The consciousness which fails to handle this stage of his development can never really handle the factors of space and time; the reality of life is limited.

The third stage, postconception, covers the period of time from conception to about the nineteenth week, halfway through development, the quickening stage, the incoming of the spirit. Here, inhibiting influences produce immaturity of character on the mental level and weakness of the upper part of the body, the chest, on the physical. During the fourth stage, which starts at the quickening, the consciousness changes from its own development to the objective world around it, and the embryo begins to move, to explore his body and his environment. It is during this stage that the very real attitudes of the mind are formed, and, if there are blocks, the child will suffer from procrastination, fear, the lack of will to go forward, and the inability to move into a situation and complete it; he will show signs of reluctance to emerge from the womb. Largely, it is the child, not the mother, who makes the act of birth difficult and painful. Tension at this stage affects the organs of the lower body, and it is here that lower back trouble begins.

Of the fifth stage, St. John wrote:

> The fifth and final stage is that of birth. Birth is the fulfilment of all that has gone before. The initial reluctance of the first stage, the challenge of the second stage, the development of the third stage, the attitudes of mind of the fourth stage, all contribute to the ability to complete this final fulfilment of entry into the outer world. The baby is a consciousness formed by the characteristics foregathered at conception and developed during gestation into a living being.

Because of these blocks in the energy flow, a child, instead of experiencing an even development, can become "stuck in time." The change in focus from the physical structure to the concept of time was one of St. John's insights and introduced a new element into healing. St. John saw that in this work the idea of physical structure can be secondary to that of time. "Time is action or change. As long as man is moving through time he is ostensibly healthy. Inasmuch as he is stuck in time he is unhealthy. This means holding on to any moment, be it five minutes or many ages ago, and not being able to move out of it."

What then is the nature of these blocks, and what creates them in the first place? Part of the answer lies in the importance of the moment of conception,

> when every single factor that decides the nature of the new person is present; a really vital and healthy pattern of factors can overcome the most injurious prenatal influences, whilst a really bad pattern can cause the new life to succumb to the mildest of influences. If there is absolutely no stress . . . the consciousness can progress through its development without conflict; but if there is any form of stress the patterns of inhibition begin to develop.

Among such stresses would be the environment of the mother at the time of conception; shock, trauma, illness; medical drugs, resentment, an adverse relationship with the father, and so on. St. John writes,

> There is another way of looking at this pattern of the blocking of the different stages of the gestation period. There are three primary actions which we use all the time in the conducting of our lives, thinking, doing and going. We use all three almost simultaneously; the first has its center in the head, the second in the thorax, shoulders and arms, the third in the pelvis and legs.

In prenatal therapy we work first on the feet, the extensions of the moving center, then on the hands and the head.

> If any of these three functions—the thinking, doing or going—is inhibited or blocked, the whole pattern of life in action is interfered with. And yet, almost without exception, we are all suffering from some form of inhibition in this way. The actions of many people are without thought or inspiration . . . others lack a true executive ability from within themselves, they function automatically. Finally, the capacity for action is lacking in a large proportion of people today, producing lethargy and inertia."

The feet are the channel through which the action of the body and the mind expresses itself. . . . Beneath the surface of all that we do is a level of inaction, and resistance to action, that produces conflict and tension in what we are doing. It is in the foot reflexes that this pattern of resistance has its expression. By working on the reflexes we are releasing the primary pattern of tensions and stresses.

We are very apt to regard this treatment as something for those who are ill; but when we change our point of view about illness and see it as a blockage, we can also see that the ostensibly normal person who is, for the moment, behaving thoroughly badly, is also suffering from a temporary blockage in his balance of life.

GASTON ST. PIERRE

Gaston St. Pierre, a practitioner and a colleague of St. John, was treating an eleven-year-old mongoloid girl who had suffered such severe brain damage at birth that leading pediatricians had predicted she would never be able to see, hear, walk, or talk. After working with her for some time, St. Pierre noticed that the attitudes of her parents and the grandfather who lived with them were undergoing subtle changes, and he recalled St. John saying that this treatment appears to bring about changes in the genetic structure. It occurred to him that, perhaps through empathy, the change is reflected in the genetic structure of the parents. He began to work on their feet, and soon he was aware of more rapid progress in the child.

One day, as St. Pierre was working on the child's right foot—the practice is to begin with the right—the child pulled it away and pushed the left foot to him. With the uncanny insight of retarded children, she understood that in the right foot are the patterns that the energy is actually working on, while the left foot holds those that are still dormant. For the next three months, she indicated that he was to work first on her left foot. Aware that her own progress was going well, she wanted to make sure that her main energies were directed to the awakening of the patterns that were still dormant.

Gaston St. Pierre's work is mostly with adults and parents. He has come to realize that the best practitioner for a child, normal or retarded, is the parent; since each parent has passed on a part of the child's genetic pattern, the parent will have an inner knowledge of when the pattern came into being. The parent will also sense how to apply the massage, within the structure of this work, so that the child's life principle can best set about restoring the primary pattern. The treatment is so simple that some parents find it hard to believe that it really works. St. John says, "The only evidence is in the result, and this is something strikingly different from that achieved by other forms of treatment given to retarded children."

Our feet are the channels of communication with the earth; the direction of our heads is toward the heavens. In the feet that the patient entrusts to our hands, memories lie buried of all time and all experience. The feet hold the key to the healing of the body and the restoration of balance to the mind. In them, we find the basic pattern of man's structure, created from the substance of earth by a Supreme Intelligence. It was not for nothing that Christ washed the feet of His disciples, linking their lives to His infinite life and blessing their whole being.

The beginning of our journey is at conception; the fulfillment is in the total realization of our humanity and our acceptance of total responsibility for what we are. This responsibility of ours is the theme of more and more important writers of today. George Leonard, in *The Silent Pulse*, writes, "The intention of the universe is evolution. Aware of it or not, each of us is involved in the grand enterprise of evolution. Our choice is whether to take responsibility. To influence the future consciously, taking responsibility for this influence, is to participate in the ultimate adventure."

29

Clearing Negative Influences from the Mind

EDWARD JASTRAM

Requirements for holism include mental health near the head of the list. An important consideration for mental health is clear communication back and forth between the conscious mind and the subconscious mind. This communication should operate with minimum obstruction and without false, alien, or "noise" signals.

To reiterate: A large proportion of our ills are said to be psychosomatic. This could mean that physical and mental operations are receiving inappropriate signals from the body/brain/mind. We can postulate that, for health, there should be good communication and positive communication among the components of mental processes. For the present examination, we will include among such components sensory apparatus and conditions, stored programs, and the superconscious, conscious, and subconscious minds. The latter may also be described as *altered states of consciousness*.

THE VARIOUS STATES OF CONSCIOUSNESS

States of consciousness, as examined by Tart[1] and others, have been defined roughly as accompanying the fundamental EEG brainwave frequency bands called beta, alpha, theta, and delta (see Figure 1).

Some of the operational characteristics of these states of consciousness follow:

234

Beta, which corresponds to conscious mind, is the frequency band
for the activities associated with normal waking consciousness,
exercise of will, the critical faculty, judgment, etc.

Alpha, Theta, and Delta, normally associated with sleep, are
called collectively the subconscious.

Alpha is also the area of dreams, rapid eye movement, creativity,
problem-solving, healing, meditation, etc.

Theta is the area exhibiting super-strength, the control of pain, the
control of bleeding, etc.

Delta is less well understood. It may be the condition for out-of-
body experience, etc.

Again, the subconscious, alpha, theta, and delta, seem to be the
area for memory, various stored positive and negative programs
such as guilt, skills, and habit, extra-sensory perception (ESP), and
what we generally call "psychic functioning."

The double line across the diagram between beta and alpha sig-

Cycles per Second					
30					
14	BETA	Normal Awake Consciousness Decision Critical Faculty			Conscious
10½	ALPHA	Dreams—R.E.M. Creativity Problem-Solving Healing	Meditation	Memory: Positive and Negative Programs— Guilt Skills Habit	Subconscious ESP Psychic Functioning "Altered States of Consciousness"
7					
4	THETA	Super-Strength Stop Pain Stop Bleeding			
½	DELTA				

Figure 1. Brain Wave Frequency Chart

nifies the separation of the conscious from the subconscious and the relative difficulty of communication, certainly at the conscious level, between the two. We might, at this point, remember that William James is quoted as saying, around the turn of the century, that "the discovery of the subconscious mind is the greatest discovery of mankind." He may well have understood that our ability to solve problems, our creativity, our health, and our ability in general to become holistic persons depend upon good communication with and through the subconscious mind.

BARRIERS, OR INTERFERENCE FACTORS

It does appear that when communication between conscious and subconscious is interfered with by various barriers, we become less able to function holistically. Such barriers interfere with our problem-solving ability, our creativity, our physical and mental healing ability, our appropriate memory recall, etc. These barriers result in confusion, depression, withdrawal, "personality aberration," physical problems which turn out to be symptoms rather than diseases, and sometimes even split personalities and subpersonalities.

The experimental paradigm states that health is the normal state for mind and body, that departures from health are brought about by barriers or interference factors, and that, upon the removal of the barriers or interference factors, the normal trend toward health of the organism will be reestablished. Further, a potent cause of departure from health in both body and mind is interference with normal conscious-subconscious communication. We examine some possible interference factors as follows:

1. Additional (alien) personalities, or "entities"
2. Obsessions, which can sometimes be described as thought-forms that can exhibit operational elements usually ascribed to "personalities"
3. Negative programs, which may be in the memory system of the subconscious, or may be associated with the Chakras (portals where energy is said to enter the body)
4. Others yet to be identified

Alien Personalities

The occurrence of additional (alien) personalities is especially important as a cause of mental disturbance. In addition, they may give rise to physical problems in the body. The concept, of course, is controversial, but the experimental results to date by people working in this field are encouraging.

Often enough, the presence of additional personalities or entities is described in terms of "split personality" or "subpersonality" of the afflicted person. In those cases which have come to attention, the problem so identified, as well as many other personality problems, have turned out to be caused by one or more alien entities or personalities which are visiting the host and which may be partially integrated into the personality of the host.

Historically, this phenomenon has been called possession and is usually thought of in terms of possession by demons or evil spirits, with intimations that the devil himself has some part in the game. There is no evidence in the work so far to support this view; rather, the words ascribed to Jesus of Nazareth, that these are "unclean spirits," come closer to the mark.

The effects of visitation by entities are many and varied, for they tend to bring their own physical and personality problems with them as well as to cause confusion by their very presence. The latter effort is the "too many cooks in the kitchen" syndrome. One may suspect the presence of entities as a probable cause of sudden personality change. Jane may say, "Since John came home from the hospital after that awful operation, I hardly know him—he's a different person." Entities may cause confusion, depression, inability to function creatively, withdrawal—many symptoms commonly described as schizoid. Since one of the primary characteristics of entities is fear, they bring fear with them and stir up latent fear programs in the host.

The overall effect or influence of the entity (or entities—one can have any number "on board") may vary from very slight to occasional complete takeover of the host; suddenly, you realize you're talking to "a different person." Usually, the effect is mild, but it can be intensified by stress.

Under what conditions may the entities come "on board"? The evidence available indicates that they attach themselves to the host personality on occasions of stress.[2] In other words, severe physical and/or mental trauma, whether induced by disease, accident, drugs, conditions of life, or other, may open the way for invasion. Any drugs are suspect, including alcohol, but, in particular, the hallucinogens appear to be open invitations to invasion. How many "bad trips" got that way because of invasion?

Who or what are these entities, and where do they come from? In our culture, persons are not very well educated or prepared for death, as Elizabeth Kübler-Ross has found.[3] The fortunate ones find it to be a pleasant experience, a "graduation" indeed. Less fortunate people, depending largely on their expectations ("You get what you expect."), find that death leaves them still functioning as personalities but without an "earth-suit" to function in, and they think they cannot function without one.[4] So they seek entrance to any earth-suit that's handy and still operating which may be open to them. The results of such invasion for the host can be confusing, to say the least. Since the invasion affects primarily the subconscious mind, the host may have little or no awareness of what's going on. If the host is aware of new problems and difficulties, he will normally not be aware of the cause.

Obsessions, or "Thought-Forms"

Other forms of invasion may be described as obsessions which, if energetic and structured enough, may be called "thought-forms" in that they take on certain aspects of personality and may be treated as such. That is to say, they appear to show initiative and purpose in a limited way, and they can cause confusion and problems of the mind and body as entities can. Obsessions and thought-forms were brought to light as possible parts of the problem when it was found that eliminating invading entities did not always solve the problems of the host.

Negative Programs

The third category, which we call negative programs in the subconscious, is made up of such influences as feelings of guilt, inferiority, inadequacy, poor self-image, negative world-perception, and fear. Some of these negative programs are said to be "in the subconscious"; others have been identified as "in the Chakras."

All of these factors, whether they be visiting entities, thought-forms, obsessions, or negative programs, produce in common the very negative result of obscuring communication back and forth between the conscious mind and the unconscious mind. This obscurity is depressing to the native (host) personality; it just doesn't function very well under these conditions. One feels cut off from one's springs of inspiration, creativity, and problem-solving. One's efficiency as an operating organism is reduced; one has lost touch with one's source. This condition is quite the opposite of holism; it is accompanied by internal stress which cannot be resolved by the host, and it can produce various chronic symptoms in the mind and in the body.[5]

Given the possibility of these negative influences, the next problem is to detect them and then clear them. Detection of the presence of entities can be accomplished in different ways, depending upon individual skills. Some people are able to "see" or visualize them, some can sense their presence, some can detect and "measure" them by dowsing as with a pendulum;[6] there may be other methods. In any event, it is desirable in dealing with this problem to be able to define what the negative influences are, how many are present, and the relative intensity of their influence on the conscious and subconscious aspects of personality.

THE CLEARING OF ENTITIES, OBSESSIONS AND OTHER PROGRAMS

No agreed upon "best way" to handle the clearing of entities, obsessions, thought-forms, and negative programs from the afflicted subject has yet emerged from the experimental work in progress. Each psychic who has become proficient in this art works within the framework of his own training, experience, and belief system, and all seem to be effective. In general, once the problem is comprehended and defined, the psychic issues mental orders as to the disposition of the entities, etc. This can be accomplished by visualization techniques, picturing mentally the end result desired, and perhaps specifying the process of accomplishing it.[7] Further visualization may be used to project energy to bring about the specified result.

The results obtained by the clearing process range all the way from quite mild to quite significant, depending mostly upon how much of the subject's problem was caused by entities. Entities can be cleared in a few minutes' time; if the problem was caused by the entities' influence only, then the problem disappears also. If additional factors, such as obsessions and negative programs, are present, it generally takes a longer period, weeks and possibly months, to clear and "ventilate" them. In a few cases, perhaps 10 to 15 percent, the procedure seems ineffective, even though the entities and programs are removed.

It is interesting to note that, in many instances, the subject knows nothing about the clearing being applied to him, so that awareness by him of suggestion plays no part in the results obtained.

For instance, a man attempted suicide as a result of deep, continued depression. Two days later, while he was still in hospital, clearing was applied in absentia, without his knowledge. The following morning, his attitude had completely changed to a positive outlook on life.

In another case, a woman who had a responsible administrative job in a technically oriented concern found herself becoming quite confused and disoriented. One evening, clearing was applied, again in absentia, and the following morning she was "back to normal."

The question has been raised as to the prevalence of the entity invasion problem. The answer from William J. Finch,[8] who has worked in this area for many years, is that perhaps 25 percent of the population seems to have this problem. My own experience would indicate that the proportion is at least that high and that many of the physical and mental difficulties coming to the attention of the medical profession, particularly the chronic ones, may be related to by this phenomenon.

BRAIN/MIND AS A COMPUTER

As a convenient framework for developing methods of working with these problems in the future, we might use the comparison of brain/mind to a computer. For instance, Dr. John Lilly[9] makes the point that we may be nothing but our programs. The analogy seems inexact, but may be useful operationally as a method of considering alternative concepts.

To begin, let us say that the whole mind (the brain, the nervous system, the various sensors, and quite probably other "operators") acts as a computer. This computer has software (programs)

CLEARING NEGATIVE INFLUENCES FROM THE MIND

of various kinds, however obtained, and it has terminals whereby access may be had to insert information, activate programs, initiate new programs, and eliminate programs already present. The conscious personality may be considered to control such a terminal, through which, presumably, it has control of the computer.

We may well inquire, however, as to the extent of the control exerted by or even available to the conscious mind at its terminal. May there be other terminals of which it is not aware? Are there programs stored in the computer quite unknown to the "operator"? Are there even "active networks" within the computer which can insert information and initiate programs apart from the volition of the "operator"?

Many of our programs are automatic, for the most part beneficial, and need no monitoring by the conscious personality. However, it appears that there can be unknown programs in the computer which are quite negative; that there can be active networks such as visiting entities, thought-forms, etc., which insert information and initiate programs in opposition to the well-being of the host; and that there is the possibility of terminals with access to the computer of which the host is unaware.

Various methods of psychic analysis of problems and psychic synthesis of solutions for them, now operational at the experimental level, offer promise. One of the reasons is that these methods attempt to address the holistic person, physical, mental, and spiritual, without limits. It is hoped that ongoing development work will lead to acceptance and usage of efficient methods which for now must be labeled unorthodox.

30

Applied Kinesiology: The Sensing and Healing Touch

JOHN F. THIE

Applied kinesiology is an outgrowth of the theory and practice of chiropractic. The theory of chiropractic is that health comes from within. People who have good posture, with the body parts relating properly one to another, have good health. The chiropractor believes that the innate intelligence that runs the body is connected to the universal intelligence that runs the world, so that each person is plugged into the universal intelligence through the nervous system. It is the job of the chiropractor to help this communication system, to insure that the body will function. He does this by working with the spine, the central core of the nervous system, the master system of the body. Then the body can take care of itself because there is no interference between the intelligences and the body.

In the early part of the 1960s, Dr. George J. Goodheart made a discovery in his private practice of chiropractic that seemed so elementary and fundamental to the manipulative practie of healing that he felt it was necessary for him to share this information with others. This discovery was that what appeared to be muscle spasm was not an overly tight, pathologically contracted muscle,

Note to reader: The alternative methods presented in this chapter are not intended to be a panacea for all health problems. They are not an attempt to keep people away from doctors, drugs, or surgery whenever they need them. Applied kinesiology can prevent some of the *needless* surgery and medication that is given for the sole purpose of satisfying the demand that something must be done when a symptom is present.

but a normal muscle that did not have opposing muscles doing the necessary counter-pull. By examining the patient for the inhibited muscle function, and directing the treatment to that correction, he could make rapid change in the body posture. Goodheart gave the name *applied kinesiology* to this approach of examining the body to determine muscle inhibition. He added a visual and mechanical technique to the practice of chiropractic, which seemed to prove, with testing of the patient, that what the chiropractors and osteopaths had been doing for 100 years with good clinical results could now be demonstrated readily to the patient and doctor.

When the muscle balance was restored, improvement in the clinical picture often occurred simultaneously. The reaction of the patient to knowing that his body was responding in a very rapid way, from methods that were unsuspected prior to this time, caused great enthusiasm on the part of both the practitioners and the patients. Patients with intractable frozen shoulders, chronic sciaticas, paralyses and other difficult situations in the musculoskeletal conditions of the body and other organ systems, seemed to get almost miraculous results. Goodheart, in his enthusiasm to share this knowledge, accepted speaking engagements from coast to coast at state and national conventions and special seminars sponsored by chiropractic organizations.

As the success of the workshop method grew, more workshops given by chiropractors for the teaching of other chiropractors grew, and Goodheart encouraged this development by naming study group leaders in various areas, so persons interested could learn the material that he had originally presented. The first meeting in 1973 was a great success, and another meeting was planned for the summer of 1974, which was also held. At that meeting, plans were begun to make the organization formal. The name International College of Applied Kinesiology was chosen, and ideas regarding its structure were presented.

FUNDAMENTALS OF APPLIED KINESIOLOGY

Man is a structural, chemical, and spiritual or psychological being, and there must be a balance among the three. The methods presented here touch on all three aspects, but the emphasis is more on the structural, since this seems to be the most neglected area. We will discuss testing, touching, and massaging the body and the muscles, using their functions, their relative strength and weakness, and the way they work in the body to get the body into better balance. This is a start toward concentrating on man's health and how to maintain it, rather than on illness and how to cure it.

MUSCLE TESTING

Testing the functions of the muscles themselves is one of the most effective ways of evaluating the structural balance we are trying to achieve. Just prior to the pain and malfunction, there are signs and symptoms which can be recognized. One of these is a weakening of the muscles and a change in the posture. If there is a tight muscle in the hip, for instance, from a corresponding weakness on the opposite side, then that hip is favored because of the tension restricting its motion. That puts a different strain on the foot, and, with the foot in a different position, there will be a strain on other sets of muscles. This is going to change the body's general posture, affecting the positions of the internal organs. That, in turn, restricts the nutrition to the organs and changes the excretions and hormonal functions. The chemical/psychological balance of the person is changed, and this affects the individual cells in the body. As the body and mind are affected, the person will think and feel differently, thereby assuming still a different posture. Then there is one more tight area, one more tension, one more cycle. Everything we do affects all the rest.

Testing the muscles performs many functions. First, it gives us an indication of the area which should be worked on. It is also a necessary part of the treatment itself. Unless a muscle has just been used, as in the tests, energies released in treatment have only a general effect throughout the body and do not always give enough benefit to the specific muscle in need of stimulation. Using the muscle first seems to tell the energies where to go and what to do.

It is also necessary to retest once the muscle has been treated. This is done for two reasons. First, the retest checks the effectiveness of the treatment. But, perhaps more important, the retest uses this muscle which has just been given a greater potential strength. While the weakness was present, the body had to compensate in order to maintain an internal balance or homeostasis. Now that the muscle has regained its strength, it is important to use it to help realign the body to a more normal position. It is the muscles which are responsible for maintaining the normal structural balance, and, unless they have been brought back into play, even though they may now be capable of being used, the body does not benefit from the muscle balancing. So first we test as an indication of the need for treatment and to give the treatment somewhere to go, and then, after treatment, we retest to help the body achieve the posture we are striving for.

The body is a whole which includes many different systems and functions, so it helps to remember that we are not just treating muscles. A problem may exist in any part of some area, and disturbances in the other systems may represent the body's efforts to compensate for the troubled system. Some of the muscles are more related to a specific organ because they may share a lymph vessel or an acupuncture meridian, for example. When we have improved the muscle by restoring the energy flow of these systems, this also gives relief to the organ which is sharing that system.

NEUROLYMPHATIC MASSAGE POINTS

While the blood stream operates under pressure, up and down in a closed circuit, the lymphatic system flows only in one direction. The lymph eventually comes to the neck region and from there empties into veins leading to the heart. The lymphatics act as a drainage system of the body, and lymph also carries proteins, hormones, and fats to all the cells. It produces antibodies within the body and makes one-quarter of the white blood cells. There are twice as many lymph vessels as there are blood vessels in the body, and twice as much lymph as blood.

The energy to the lymphatic system is regulated by what we call neurolymphatic reflexes, located mainly on the chest and back. These reflex points act like circuit breakers or switches that get turned off when the system is overloaded. The location of the reflex points does not seem to correspond to the positions of the lymph glands, but they are related.

The neurolymphatic points vary in size from a little pellet to a small bean, and they occur either alone or in groups, sometimes scattered over an entire muscle. Some can be felt, and others cannot. They are usually tender spots, and the tenderness is usually greater in the front of the body than in the back. The reflexes or areas which are found to be the most sore seem to be the ones in greatest need of deep massage. Once the reflexes have been turned on in this way, the blockage in the energy of the lymph flow to the organ and muscle is relieved, and the weak muscle will have improved in strength when retested.

NEUROVASCULAR HOLDING POINTS

Neurovascular holding points are located mainly on the head. For strengthening a muscle, these points require simple contact with the pads of the fingers, merely touching and slightly stretching the skin. A few seconds after contact is made, a slight pulse can be felt at a steady rate of seventy to seventy-four beats per minute. This pulse is not related to the heartbeat, but is believed to be the primitive pulsation of the microscopic capillary bed in the skin. After a pulse has been felt on both sides and it has become synchronized, then the neurovascular points may be held for about twenty seconds or up to ten minutes, depending on the severity of the problem. This appears to improve the blood circulation to both the muscle and the related organ, and the weak muscle will have increased in strength when retested.

ACUPUNCTURE AND ACUPRESSURE

There is a great similarity between the Chinese health philosophy and the philosophy of chiropractic. Oriental acupuncturists are now coming to the Western chiropractic colleges, and they, too, are finding great similarities between the two methods of healing. In China, the traditional treatment of the acupuncture meridians is to use fine needles or slivers of bamboo to stimulate the areas. In Russia, France, Japan, and China many doctors stimulate these same points by massage and touching.

Acupressure vessels, or meridians, are located throughout the body. They contain a free-flowing, colorless, noncellular liquid which may be partly actuated by the heart. These meridians have been measured and mapped by modern technological methods, electronically, thermically, and radioactively. With practice, they can also be felt. There are specific acupuncture points along the meridians. These points are electromagnetic in character and consist of small, oval cells called bonham corpuscles which surround the capillaries in the skin, the blood vessels, and the organs throughout the body. There are some 500 points which are being used both with needles and massage, depending on the action desired.

CEREBROSPINAL FLUID

The flow of cerebrospinal fluid is believed to be affected by the almost microscopic movement of the cranial bones during breathing. If these bones in the skull become slightly stuck together, then it appears that the fluid is not pumped well enough through the spinal column. This can cause weakness in the muscles, since the energy related to the cerebrospinal fluid is not flowing freely. Adjustment of the cranial bones is a difficult technique which should be reserved for doctors, but there is one simple technique which lay people can use. When the abdominal muscles are weak, this is often due to the parietal bones being jammed together at the top of the head. Pulling apart on the skull along the seam, as if to split the scalp along a middle part, using hard pressure, is very effective in strengthening the abdominals.

OTHER PEOPLE USING APPLIED KINESIOLOGY

Up until now, most of these methods and techniques have been exclusively the province of the chiropractic profession. Now, however, many other helping professionals are finding applied kinesiology useful when practiced in conjunction with their own specialties. Following are just a few.

Robert Riddler, D.C., in the Seattle area, developed a method of testing vitamins using muscle-testing and has gone on to innovate other ways to use muscle-testing.

Herman Stoffels, D.C., in Northern California, has taken the Riddler technique and branched off yet another way to use applied kinesiology. He calls it *test response technique.*

Robert Peshek, D.D.S., further developed the muscle-testing for nutritional substances and wrote *Balancing Body Chemistry with Nutrition.*

George Eversaul, Ph.D., in Las Vegas, is a biofeedback expert who has developed a way to use applied kinesiology in dentistry.

Called *dental kinesiology,* this specialty relates nutrition and the position of the teeth to muscle weakness throughout the body.

John Diamond, M.D., trained as a psychiatrist in Australia, now lives in New York. When he learned about applied kinesiology, he gave up his psychiatric practice and went to study with Dr. Goodheart and others and has now developed a new area called *behavioral kinesiology* which uses muscle-testing.

"TOUCH FOR HEALTH"—APPLIED KINESIOLOGY FOR LAY PEOPLE

We now know that these methods of health enhancement are not harmful and that lay people can use them to help each other without endangering themselves or others.

Touch for Health is an educational system whose purpose is to give the general public some of the safe, simple, easy-to-use techniques which have been developed in the last fifteen years in chiropractic, together with the modern practice of ancient disciplines and knowledge of Oriental health management. By learning to listen to and feel what is going on in our bodies, we are able to correct the minor problems before they develop into serious illnesses. Using the methods of applied kinesiology as taught in *Touch for Health* will help prevent malfunctions and pains from developing, as well as correct the reason for the pain and allow the life force to flow uninterrupted through the body.

Many of the ways to help the body function more fully require a second person. For example, it is very difficult to test one's own muscle, which is the primary tool of assessment. *Touch for Health* principles used between family members can help foster communication and trust as they begin to help each other toward a feeling of health and vitality.

31

A Bird's-Eye View of Oriental Medicine

MARC ESTRIN

As 800 million Chinese turn their heads toward Ford and Coca-Cola, we in the West are—in our turn—turning East. The sixties saw the youth culture embrace a panoply of Eastern religions; a decade later, Nixon, a bizarre Marco Polo, opened the trade routes, and all at once the myriad phenomena of a five-millennia-old culture blossomed forth, ripe for the Western media and the ever-hungry mass mind.

One of the "wonders of the East" to attract attention earliest was the science of acupuncture. As an amazed public gaped at films of fully conscious patients under acupuncture anesthesia on operating tables, suffering no pain, delegations of skeptical doctors trooped over to China to "check it out." They brought back miracle stories, but little understanding of an ancient, pragmatic, healing art. Their colleagues at home remained dubious and suspicious, but not so the public. Rumors circulated of curing the previously incurable, of avoiding surgery, of inexpensive, do-it-yourself treatments. To a nation so concerned with its own poor health as ours, such news was good news indeed. But with few or no practitioners available, traditional Oriental medicine remained a vague possibility, vaguely sensed by the multitudes and vaguely acknowledged by the medical establishment.

Until quite recently. In the last two or three years, a kind of critical mass has been reached. Eastern ways of health and healing are being increasingly accepted in the West. Native practitioners are being trained, and are introducing the public to the realities and the limits of this old, new medicine. And, transplanted to new soil, ancient traditions are being transformed, as they themselves transform their participants.

THE UNIQUE PRINCIPLE

All aspects of Far Eastern philosophy are based on one principle, which is symbolically represented in Figure 1. The figure is contained within a circle representing undifferentiated infinity. This circle is divided into a dark side (*yin*) and a light side (*yang*)—opposing, but complementary elements.* Yin and yang are not, however, merely in opposition, but are interfaced in a sinuous curve, a frozen undulation (contrast with Figure 2). This implies that in the infinite universe, yin and yang are eternally fluctuating, and that all things partake of varying quantities of each. Nothing is all yin; nothing is all yang. At the extremes, yang tends to change into yin, yin into yang.

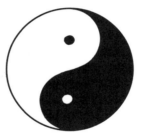

Figure 1. The T'ai Chi, or Great Origin

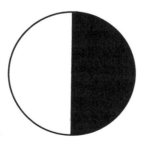

Figure 2. Dark and Light in Simple Opposition

* Yin may be symbolized by ∇, yang by △, their balance by ✡.

But that is not all. At the center of the darkness is a spot of light, and at the center of the light, an equal spot of darkness (see Figure 1). This represents a fundamental observation: everything contains the seed of its opposite. At the height of summer, June 21, the days begin to grow shorter. In the dead of winter, hidden life under the snow gathers itself toward growth. Thus, the relationship of yin and yang is subtle and all-pervasive, as depicted by the T'ai Chi. And the depiction is only a two-dimensional representation of a sphere of infinite radius; all of us, swirling and embracing, are within.

YIN AND YANG, AND CHI FLOW

What are yin and yang in the real world? The perspicacious eye can see them interacting in all phenomena: positive and negative, day and night, male and female.

The fundamental difference from which all others flow is that yin is expansive, yang contractive. Between them, they generate the pulsation and breathing of the universe. In the daytime— bright, warm, yang—things contract and are sharply defined and rational. But at night—dark, cool, yin—expansion, mystery, and intuition reign.

Nothing is all yin or all yang; the healthy male has female within and vice versa, at the personal, psychological, hormonal, and archetypal levels. Night changes to day; it is darkest and coldest just before dawn. The light of the stars (yang) is visible only in the dark (yin). Our inactivity in sleep (yin) allows the intense activity (yang) of our dream life.

Each of these antinomies creates a tension between its complementary, antagonistic elements. The sum total of all these turbulent stretches and interactions is the T'ai Chi. The collective negative is the yin, the collective positive, the yang.

Just as the positive and negative poles of a battery, when connected create a flow of electrons, a current, so do yin and yang create a current, a force through the world (see Figure 3). That force is called *Chi* (*Ki* in Japanese), the moving power of the universe. Chi flows through all things, nourishing them, generating from them, energy and continuity.

Examples of Yin and Yang
(adapted from Kushi, *The Book of Macrobiotics*, p. 9)

YIN	YANG
Expansion	Contraction
Diffusion	Fusion
Dispersion	Assimilation
Decomposition	Organization
More inactive and slower	More active and faster
Shorter wave and high frequency	Longer wave and low frequency
Ascent and vertical	Descent and horizontal
More outward and periphery	More inward and central
Lighter	Heavier
Colder	Hotter
Darker	Brighter
Wetter	Drier
Thinner	Thicker
Longer	Shorter
Softer	Harder
Fragile	Durable
Vegetable	Animal
Female	Male
Gentle, negative	Active, positive
Psychological and mental	Physical and social
Space	Time

HOLISTIC HEALTH

What has all this to do with health care? Simply this: the health of all things, animate and inanimate, varies with their ability to conduct Chi, balancing yin and yang in ways appropriate to their particular forms. This is the fundamental perception of Oriental medicine, a perception not included in Western science. It flows directly out of the Oriental understanding of the nature of the universe as represented by the T'ai Chi. Traditional Oriental medicine is an organic part of Eastern philosophy, organized around the all-pervading Unique Principle of the T'ai Chi. It understands man as both macro- and microcosm, of and in the Unity of the Cosmos.

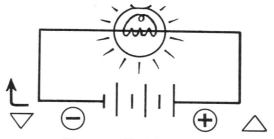

Figure 3. Chi Movement

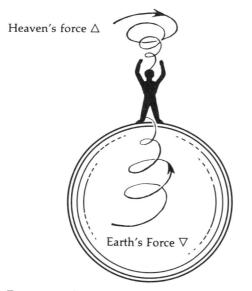

Figure 4. The Chi Flowing Through the Patient

Consequently, traditional Oriental medicine is truly holistic. It looks at the patient, not the disease, and sees her as a complex organism standing at a particular place on the planet, in a given year, at a given season, at a given time of day. All these factors affect the Chi flowing through her and the balance of yin and yang. Heaven's force (yang) flows down from above; Earth's force (yin) up from below (see Fig. 5). The quality of the individual's physical organism will determine whether these forces flow freely throughout the body, sustaining good health, or become congested or imbalanced, creating disease.

CHANNELS OF CHI FLOW

Chi flows through the body in paths called meridians. Ancient man, before recorded history, must have discovered that rubbing certain places on the body created predictable effects. As more and more of these points were found, together with ways and combinations in which to stimulate them, a detailed map began to grow, and patterns to appear. Finally, in a kind of connect-the-dots manner, practitioners drew imaginary lines on the body relating chains of points which seemed to work in concert. These lines seemed to be the paths of energy flow, the acupuncture meridians.

Traditionally, there were twelve such meridians, six connecting the upper limbs with the torso, six connecting the lower. Two additional ones ran up the midline, front and back, making fourteen in all. People realized that these were probably not the only such meridians, but only those containing points on the surface of the body through which the energy flow could be conveniently manipulated. Internally, out of reach of thumb or needle, were likely to be hundreds of other paths, all interconnected with the fourteen and with each other. Indeed, certain breathing and psychic exercises are directed at these unknown, but hypothesized channels.

These treatment maps, along with other ancient knowledge of medical practice, were handed down and preserved in oral tradition, and finally in written form, in the *Nei Ching, The Yellow Emperor's Classic of Internal Medicine,* around the fourth century B.C.

Acupuncture, acupressure and moxibustion are three methods developed to manipulate Chi flow. The first uses needles, the second, the fingers, and the third, minute application of heat to stimulate the traditional points for a desired effect. The choice and uses of these methods—which points, in what combinations, to be used for what—are the content of the practitioner's art.

FIVE-ELEMENT THEORY

For each method, the available points are the same: the traditional acupuncture points on the traditional acupuncture meridians. The theory of their combination and use is also the same: the acupuncturist utilizes a small part of an all-encompassing picture, that of *five-element theory.*

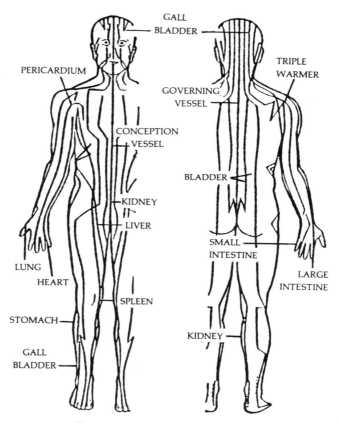

Figure 5. Channels of Chi Flow

Five-element theory is the basis of the practical level of the Unique Principle. It relates all phenomena in a cyclical continuum of yin and yang.

The five traditional elements are not meant to be taken literally, but as symbols for relative states of yin/yang composition and their transformations. Thus, metal represents the most densified, solid state (yang). Water represents melting or decomposing (liquid), while wood contains the idea of going up from the earth, expanding. Fire is the extreme yin part of the cycle which, by its very action, creates the condensing ashes of earth. We can see the whole cycle in operation in the commonly observed states of water:

Metal state = ice
Water state = common water
Wood state = starting to evaporate
Fire state = dispersed vapor
Earth state = condensing vapor, clouds

What makes this concept powerful are the relations among the various parts of the circle. The external cycle, reading clockwise around the pentagon, is the creative, or mother-daughter cycle. Each element gives birth to, and nourishes, the next in line. Water creates and feeds wood; wood, fire; fire, earth; and so on. Proceeding in the reverse direction, however, we find an over-nourished child harming its parent, as too much fire will burn wood and too much soil will put out fire.

The inner star shows the destructive cycle. Water will extinguish fire, fire will melt metal, metal will cut wood, etc.

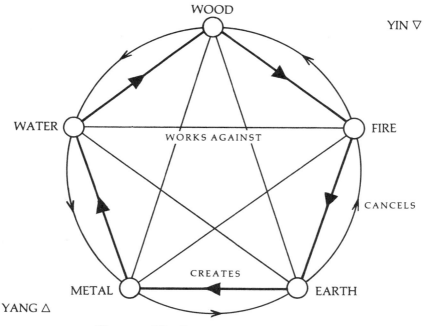

Figure 6. The Five Traditional Elements

Relating the Five Elements to Other Factors
(from M. Kushi lecture notes)

	WOOD	FIRE	EARTH	METAL	WATER
solid organs	liver	heart	spleen/ pancreas	lungs	kidney
hollow organs	gall bladder	small intestine	stomach	large intestine	bladder
senses	sight	taste	touch	smell	hearing
direction	east	south	center	west	north
season	spring	early summer	late summer	autumn	winter
colors	blue	red	yellow	white	black
tastes	sour	bitter	sweet	spicy	salty
weather	windy	hot	humid	dry	cold
emotions	anger	laughter	thinking	worry	fear
voices	shouting	talking	singing	crying	groaning
grains	wheat	corn	millet	rice	beans
fruits	plum	apricot	date	peach	chestnut

Let's look at an example of how this might be used to make therapy decisions. Suppose a patient were having digestive problems due to a weak stomach, say, putting out insufficient acid. Our first thought might be to stimulate his stomach meridian. Consulting the above chart, we see that the stomach is an "earth" organ. Stimulating it would be fine if there were also weakness, say, in the lungs or large intestine (metal), its daughters. These, too, would be strengthened thereby. But suppose the patient also had a weak kidney, a weak "water" organ. Stimulating the stomach would have a destructive effect, further weakening the kidney—as can be seen on the inner star. A better approach, then, would be to stimulate the "fire" organs (heart or small intestine) and allow the mother/daughter effect to strengthen the stomach without weakening the kidney.

Such considerations, elementary from an Oriental point of view, are beyond the scope of Western medicine. Who knows how many "complications" have needlessly occurred for lack of them?

The relationships shown in Figure 7 yield many other interesting results. Suppose a patient were suffering many stress-related symptoms due to worry. Since worry is a "metal" emotion, our strategy might be to increase all the "fire" inputs we could. In addition to stimulating the heart, heart governer, small intestine, and triple warmer meridians, we might consider dressing the patient in red, or increasing his consumption of bitter foods. We might make sure he is warmly dressed, and keep him laughing. We could buttress these tactics (assuming none were contraindicated by other considerations) by using reverse mother/daughter pressure from the "water" column. The experienced practitioner can bring all these factors into play in achieving his patient's cure.

If such a mix seems odd, it must be remembered that all the parameters on the chart are but expressions of yin/yang composition—the one variable crucially at work. Chi flow in the yin/yang battery can be affected by manipulating *any* of its manifestations. And, since Chi flow affects everything, imbalances can show up anywhere. These considerations can help illuminate two of the more mysterious aspects of Oriental practice, psychic healing and pulse and visual diagnosis.

PSYCHIC HEALING

Compared to a bulldozer or even a clenched fist, Chi exerts a very gentle force. It is an extremely yin phenomenon, low in amplitude, but all-pervasive. Although it can be concentrated by yogis and karate masters to produce unbelievable effects,[1] the average person deals with it much as she does with the air around her—thoughtlessly, with little effort. Yet its very softness is responsible for one of its most remarkable properties: it can be manipulated by the mind. Most minds cannot move mountains (or even bend spoons), but they *can* affect Chi flow. Consequently, Oriental medicine utilizes awareness on the part of both patient and practitioner to aid in healing.

When a good acupuncturist inserts a needle, she simultaneously pushes the energy along the sought-after path with her psyche. Neither is the patient passive. He visualizes the healing energy penetrating, flowing in the required directions. If the concentration of both is strong enough, changes can be effected without needles or touch at all. This is psychic healing. It is practiced in many cultures, and the achievements of its great masters, such as Jesus, have been recorded throughout the ages—including our own[2]—as evidence that there is more to life than meets the eye.

Western medicine acknowledges the placebo effect, but only as a somewhat dishonest red herring to be dealt with. Oriental medicine understands it, and uses it as a powerful, legitimate tool.

ORIENTAL DIAGNOSIS

While certain facets of traditional Oriental diagnosis—interrogation and palpation for painful areas—are vaguely related to Western technique, its two major aspects are completely unknown here. The first is visual diagnosis. An astute Oriental observer, armed with a deep understanding of yin and yang and its all-pervasive expression, can tell at a glance what is going on with a patient. His present condition, his past and future life, even the character of his parents can be read in his general structure and coloring, the shape of his eyes, mouth, hands, fingernails. Nothing is accidental; everything is an expression of the forces of yin and yang in his body. An imbalance within can be clearly read on the surface.[3] Interrogation is used only to confirm or modify these initial impressions.

With pulse diagnosis, the practitioner is able to determine the state of Chi flow in the acupuncture meridians. Using three fingers on the left or right radial artery, and either light or deep pressure, he can "listen" to the quality of each of the twelve pulses. After years of training and experience, he can identify as many as sixty-four different types of pulse in each meridian, the combinations yielding a detailed picture of internal states. Compare the Western practitioner who, although he considers the pulse a "vital sign," takes into account only its rate and rhythm.

By far the most important attribute of Oriental diagnosis is that

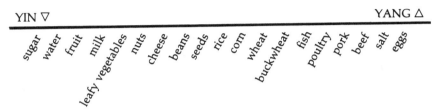

Figure 7. The Balance of Yin and Yang in Common Foods

it can be used *before symptoms develop.* In the West, a patient gets "sick" before he goes to a doctor. An Eastern practitioner, however, using the above noninvasive diagnostic methods, can pick up a deficiency or superfluity of Chi, or a yin/yang imbalance, before it results in the breakdown of related organs. Treatment is directed at adjustment, and an acute situation is avoided. Truly preventive medicine.

THE IMPORTANCE OF DIET

In Oriental medicine, proper eating is seen as the fundamental way of establishing harmony with the universe and enjoying the good health which follows.

Food, like everything else, displays a varying balance of yin and yang. Some common foods arranged on a spectrum of most yin to most yang are shown in Figure 7.

Within each category, the smaller and more condensed, the more yang; the larger and most expanded, the more yin. A smaller nut is more yang than a larger one; a larger, sweeter fruit is more yin than a more contracted one.

A healthy diet is one which balances yin and yang in a manner appropriate to environmental conditions. For example, in a hot, yang climate, it is necessary to eat in a yin manner.

According to Oriental medicine, one of the greatest health disasters of history has been the long-distance transportation of foods in a north-south direction. Animal species evolved eating local foods, and they were automatically balanced with their environment.

The traditional Oriental diet centers around the grains and vegetables in the middle of the spectrum. Such a balance is more stable, and Oriental culture is, as a result, quieter and more contemplative than our own, and more aware of the harmonious place of each being in the universe.

SOME GENERAL OBSERVATIONS

Turn East as we may, we in the West cannot simply swallow Eastern culture whole, much as it might benefit us. Too many Oriental operating principles conflict with our long-standing assumptions. There is our need for visible and measurable explanations. If either we or our instruments cannot see or measure something, we have learned to be biased against its existence. This explains why so many Western scientists do not "believe" in acupuncture, though its results can be readily seen. "If there are meridians conducting energy in the body, why can't we, with our most powerful electron microscopes, find them?"

A reasonable question. Yet, if we look at the history of science, we see that there have always been elements, at any given time, beyond its horizon.

Furthermore, if we look at the human body through T'ai Chi-colored glasses, we can see it as an arrangement of increasingly yin layers around a yang core. At the center is the hard yang skeleton. Over that, the semisolid muscle and soft-tissue layer. More yin than that, the liquid blood, and, more yin still, the electricity to the nervous system. Why not then an even more yin system, so yin as to be independent of conducting structures, using the body as a whole as a conductor, guided along its meridians by the interacting fields within?

A most interesting phenomenon is the finding of numerous contradictions about acupuncture among the Oriental experts. No two books will describe the same treatment for what appears to be the same condition. Some authors claim that the type of needle or the direction of rotation will either excite or sedate a point, while others assert that all stimulation is normative, bringing up a lack of energy or calming down an excess. One world-famous British expert, Felix Mann, claims that one needn't stimulate points accurately at all—that a needle anywhere within a large "zone" will be effective.

A most serious controversy involves the traditional school of acupuncture, which insists that the lefthand pulses of a man are equivalent to the righthand pulses of a woman and vice versa, while the "modern" school holds that the position of the male and female pulses are the same. All pulse diagnosis hangs on this.

The only way I have been able to come to grips with these contradictions is to assume that all the experts are right, and that their techniques work for *them*—in part, because they and their patients believe in them. This is not quackery or placebo effect, but a clear application of the mind affecting Chi flow.

Perhaps the single most difficult aspect of our turning East is that of a materialist culture trying to incorporate a spiritual one.

There is little room in our scientific thought-world for an anatomy and physiology embracing soul and spirit. If the West is to appreciate and assimilate Oriental medicine to any significant extent, it will have to expand its current view of man and the universe.

CULTURAL, POLITICAL AND SOCIAL IMPLICATIONS

A West that could truly accept Oriental medicine would experience a new sense of awe, and its spiritual senses would be heightened. Should Oriental medicine enter our culture in an authentic way, our eating habits, and thus our habits of life and thought, would change significantly. Health would be entrusted to the individual, and the physician would be established as an educator and advisor. Symptomatic health care could be provided by mid-level practitioners and technicians, as it is done by "barefoot doctors" in modern China, and inexpensive treatments would become available for general use. The holistic health movement would be dramatically advanced.

Such changes in society always come slowly, over the determined opposition of those who are displaced or discomfited by the changes. The benefits to society appear so great, however, that such an outcome is not unthinkable.

32

Orthodox Western Medicine in the Holistic Era

PETER ALBRIGHT

An obvious question comes to the mind of the reader of holistic health subjects, especially one who has only recently come across these subjects for the first time, and that is: "What will happen to orthodox Western medicine as time goes on?" After all, aren't we saying that holistic health care will prevent a lot of illness, and doesn't this mean that eventually there will be little for traditional doctors to do?

That question has neither a simple nor an easy answer. We must attempt an answer only with great care and deliberation. First, this spills over into the area of prediction, which is hazardous unless one is truly clairvoyant! Secondly, we are sometimes tempted to simplify matters which are very complex, for the sake of making them more understandable.

It seems to me that there is one answer to the question for the near future and perhaps another for the more distant future. I expect that the ideas which make up holistic health care, such as assuming personal responsibility, developing intuition and discrimination, cancelling old programs, rebalancing energy on all levels of being, and so on, will gradually enter the lives of more and more people as their effectiveness is appreciated. Just as we have seen the salutary effects of environmental sanitation and control of malnutrition and starvation in parts of the world, we will see clearly the beneficial effects of what we now call holistic thinking and living.

We will see the incidence of many present-day problems diminishing. The scourges of today, such as cancer, heart disease, alcoholism, and traffic accidents, will go into decline, just as did plague, tuberculosis, smallpox, and polio in generations past. We are going to meet the challenges of tomorrow, just as the challenges of yesterday were met, but we will meet them with the appropriate tools.

So, the answer to the question for the near future is that we may notice only slight changes in the way orthodox medicine is practiced in the main. Then, with the passage of more time, a number of interesting things can be expected to happen.

As we have seen in the discussion of the medical model, experts are already predicting that, as early as 1990, we will be noticing excessive numbers of traditionally trained physicians, because of the post World War II expansion of medical schools. I have already referred to some of the problems expected to stem from this, but another very likely possibility is that many more physicians by that time will be developing an interest in holistic medicine. This is a trend that will be interesting to watch. After some adjustments in attitudes, the general public will undoubtedly benefit from the trend.

A BLENDING OF OLD AND NEW

Another aspect of this whole question that is interesting and important to explore is the role of what we now call traditional Western medicine in the scheme of holistic health care. Under what circumstances will people or their holistic practitioners call upon medical doctors to meet health needs?

The blending of the old and the new is a crucial issue. It is vital that all who are concerned with health care strive for this blending. As the old saying goes, we must not throw out the baby with the bath water! The great contributions of medical science in the past must be recognized, along with its potential for making great contributions in the future.

At the same time, the value of the holistic approach must, and ultimately will, be recognized by more and more people for what it is—a broadening and expanding of our scientific understanding of ourselves and our environment through multiple approaches to health and well-being, rather than what some now see as a delving into the occult, using questionable methods to arrive at conclusions which cannot be supported scientifically. We have discussed in an earlier chapter the reasons for the error of the latter conception.

We all have within us, even the newborn child with Downs syndrome, the potential for bringing about our own healing with the help of others. Knowledge of this healing gift is the larger understanding into which will eventually be integrated all of the apparently disparate approaches to well-being which are contained in both Eastern and Western traditions, which use both ancient and ultramodern methods, and which are applied on physical, mental, emotional, and spiritual levels of being.

SPECIALIZED FUNCTION

When we look at this full spectrum of health and healing, as we also did in the "Breakdown Lane," it becomes clear that the physician and nurse trained in the modern Western tradition and working primarily around the hospital model have a very special and essential function to perform in our society. That function is the highly specialized and scientific treatment of serious health breakdown. A cohort of mine in holistic health put it succinctly not long ago when she said, "If I fall off my motorcycle and break my leg, don't take me to the health food store! I want to go to the nearest hospital emergency room."

There are several kinds of health situations in which the fully trained doctor and nurse have particular expertise. They are situations which we might look forward to seeing eliminated in the very long run. But, in the meantime (and that's a long time), they are situations in which people will still find themselves, and where they will need prompt, skillful, and effective treatment.

First, there are accidents and injuries, including head injury, internal injuries, fractures, lacerations, burns, and the like. Then there are acute serious illnesses, such as appendicitis, pneumonia, intestinal obstruction, pancreatitis, heart attack, stroke, and acute bleeding. Some of these conditions are treatable in alternative ways as well, but many people prefer traditional approaches.

Then there are chronic problems, such as severe diabetes, obstructive lung disease, liver and kidney failure, and chronic heart failure, all of which are improved by careful measurement of physical and chemical factors and adjustment of the internal environment of the patient according to complicated scientific principles. Finally, there are complex clinical situations in which either the diagnosis is elusive or the patient remains ill despite all measures used to foster recovery.

COMBINING APPROACHES

Having said that these are conditions in which Western scientific medical expertise will be needed, we must also reiterate that people in all such situations have been helped by the use of alternative therapies in conjunction with the standard ones. The plea that I would make, as a person standing with one foot in the Western tradition for over a quarter century and the other now firmly in the holistic future, is that we all recognize the unique value of each kind of therapy and use the various approaches synergistically. Most therapies are compatible with each other (one learns about any others) and can safely be used in combinations. Indeed, the principle of combined therapy is used extensively within the traditional medical model, and is found to have advantages over single therapies.

So we have seen a number of ways, including traditional medicine, in which people help other people with their healing. We have touched on only a few of the many approaches which are in regular and effective use today. As we gather more and more experience with the combined use of various therapies, we will see that many more people can be helped by a broadened and enriched spectrum of healing energies.

PART V
Health and Wholeness:
The Realization
of Well-Being

33

A Gathering of Friends: The Holistic Health Center

PETER ALBRIGHT

A s people have become more and more aware of the great value of the many alternative therapies we have been discussing, and of the many more we have not had space to discuss, they have a recurring thought which just won't go away: a way must be found to organize the various skills of alternative therapists so that people can receive the maximum benefits from those abilities which exist in the community. Thus the idea of the Holistic Health Center has gradually emerged.

We are now in the first years of this process. Many centers have been organized in Britain, Western Europe, and the United States. At this stage of the process, every center differs widely from every other center. This happens, of course, whenever society is in the middle of a new learning curve. I would like to present a few thoughts arising out of my own experience of helping to plan and organize holistic centers in Vermont.

What are the most important issues raised in the process of developing a holistic health center? Not necessarily in order of importance, I have found that the following are among them:

1. *What is our purpose?* This is important to enunciate. A statement of purpose unites planners around common goals and informs the community of the group's intentions.

269

2. *What kinds of services are we going to provide?* The answer to this will be determined in part by the people who are available to provide them. One service which is a constant is education, a cornerstone of holistic health care. Another is helping the client develop a personal health maintenance program, which includes nutrition, rest and exercise balance, and a meditation or deep-relaxation method. The kinds of services which may vary in different centers will be such things as counseling, psychotherapy, massage, yoga, acupuncture, kinesiology, and many other possible combinations. A center may also have a Western-trained physician or nurse to deal with various needs, but, in many centers, this is not available.

3. *What other capabilities should we have in our center?* These may include information-gathering, referral to community resources, audit and evaluation, newsletter or journal, and the like.

4. *How are we to be organized?* This raises questions about incorporation and supervision of activities at the center. Among the issues to be faced are: Who is "in charge," how affiliated practitioners are screened and selected, how the quality of care is monitored, how the results of care are evaluated, and how referrals are made within the group.

5. *What kind of space are we going to need?* This involves consideration of educational programs as well as individual diagnosis and therapy space.

6. *Where will the money we need come from?* Among the possibilities: fees-for-services, prepayment, possibility and desirability of grants, and others.

7. *How can we maintain a good relationship with the community around us?* In addition to a newsletter, liaison with the rest of the health care community, public education programs, the question of involvement in public issues relating to health, and so on are considerations.

In my experience, it is well worth wrestling with all these issues to achieve the result: a gathering of friends linked in a special way with people who recognize a need for this kind of relationship. Practitioners who choose to unite in this way are usually already practicing successfully in other locations. But they feel that people's needs can be served better by the kinds of caring and healing relationships which the holistic health center makes possible.

I would like to speak from the heart about some things which concern me during this period when we try to conceive of a model, or models, of helping situations which will be most appropriate for a society which is moving—no, leaping—ahead in awareness.

First, I want to consider balance. If we are to help bring balance to people's lives, each of us should have achieved a certain balance in our own lives. We should have learned a great many of the lessons we would teach our students about life. There are, of course, many balances. There is a balance between youthful, bounding enthusiasm and a more placid wisdom and detachment. There is a balance between boldness and caution. There is a balance between a past which may have been disappointing and perhaps frustrating, but in which we have gained knowledge and experience, and the future of which we dream, bright and glittering but as yet untested.

In a practical sense, the idea of balance can be seen in many ways, but my thought especially pictures the gathering of friends arranged in a circle or set of intersecting circles about the distressed client, and the strength which can come from the proper balancing of those circles. What can be more "holistic" than this, as we consider how to help the client to strike a number of inner balances among the realms of body, mind, emotions, and the higher self? Only from the strength of such inner balances can the individual deal with fellow beings and the external environment in a calm and joyous way.

Another attribute which we as helpers should possess is maturity, since we wish to help our clients reach a state of mature, healthy functioning. If we live in a state of excessive emotional dependence on others to satisfy our needs, we should strive to transform that dependence into feelings of strength and self-sufficiency to the point where we are in balance with our fellow beings, but not to the point where everyone else is leaning on *us!* That would only reveal in us an excessive need to be leaned upon. Other aspects of maturity, such as patience, sound judgment, and clear thinking, also contribute mightily to a healthy group.

When the friends gather around the growing and learning client, the collective maturity of the group should be evident, so that a sense of strength, evenness, and safety can be shared with, and eventually conferred upon, the client. It is also clear that it is healthy for a group if its members do not spend an inordinate amount of time, and the group's energy, as clients working out their dependency patterns.

An equally necessary quality which a healing group of any kind should generate is a sense of cooperation—with each other, with the client, and in the world. For many people, this is a hard lesson to learn in a culture where competition is praised so highly and is always described as "healthy." But a spirit of cooperation strengthens the bonds between the healing friends and brings about the synergistic effect which embodies the holistic concept—that the whole is greater than the sum of its parts. This is true at the group level as well as at the level of the individual person.

It is becoming more and more clear to me that a sufficient amount of attention must be paid to the presence or absence of all these qualities in the members of a group dedicated to helping and healing. Many fledgling groups have failed and will fail because inadequate time and attention have been devoted to these things.

The extent to which the holistic health movement has already grown is testimony to the eagerness with which practitioners and the public alike are approaching this new form of health practice and are sensing that it has meaning for their lives. Undoubtedly, a large part of its appeal and its value is that the person at the center of all the activity is the client, who is being urged and helped to achieve both personal responsibility and higher consciousness of life, along with a sustained level of vibrant health.

*   *   *   *   *

In the following chapter, Marcus McCausland, writing from the midst of the National Health Service in England, will give us his perspective on the future of health care, placing considerable emphasis on how community resources might be organized for better health.

34

The Future of Health Care

MARCUS McCAUSLAND

I n order to think intelligently about the future of health care, we might look at some principles that have emerged from the World Health Organization in Geneva. We need to realize that these principles are emerging *because* it has become clear to concerned people that something has gone wrong with our society and that the quality of life is falling.

First, in order to change the trend, a holistic approach to health care is required. This involves deciding upon an acceptable holistic model of man before we can bring about change.

Next, health care needs to be decentralized to communities. A model is needed for a caring community where the human touch is normal in all relationships.

Then, there will be a change in the near future from a "repair" system, such as we have at the moment, to a low-cost system where the main emphasis is on the promotion of health, with secondary emphasis on the cure of illness.

Finally, there will be a gradual integration of all methods of diagnosis and therapy, and methods which may be considered unconventional at this time, will be used in conjunction with conventional methods.

We have said that, to understand holistic health care, a holistic model of man is required (see Figure 1).

The model shows a human being divided into seven aspects and illustrates how our Inner Self (or soul) relates to the world around us through six windows, through each of which there is a constant flow in and out of different forms of energy and information.

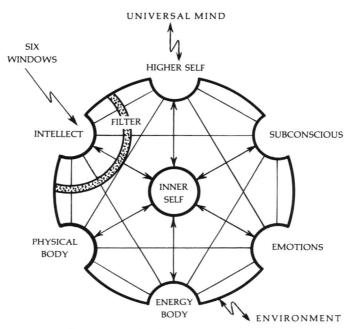

Figure 1. A Holistic Model of Man

These windows are controlled by our mind and emotions so that the amount of energy or information that we emit or admit is decided by *us*. For instance, at night, when we go to sleep, we close down our body and cover it up so that the minimum amount of energy is radiated.

We can do the same with all our other windows—either voluntarily or involuntarily. In some cases, this can lead to pain and suffering. For instance, if we are badly let down in a love affair or neglected by our parents when young, we may completely or partially close our emotional window so that we do not give or receive love. In later life, this can cause serious health problems.

The lines joining the different aspects indicate that there is a continuous interchange—a complete link—among all aspects of ourselves. If one window opens or closes, then all the other windows are directly affected for better or worse. Some examples will help to illustrate this.

If the brain is damaged in an accident, the intellectual window may close completely. The individual concerned may be in deep coma. The body will continue to run itself, like a vegetable, but the family will be unable to communicate. To all intents and purposes that human being appears to be dead. However, and this is the important aspect of this model, through love and prayer it *may* be possible to make contact with the Inner Self of that individual and to help him to find his way back to full life and health.

If an individual is deeply disturbed emotionally, the physical body will be affected. Digestion will be impaired. This will influence the flow of blood to the brain, and thus the intellect will be lowered in efficiency.

A whole being can be likened to a rainbow. When sunlight passes through raindrops, the light is broken down into its component parts. Each of the seven colors is unique, but, when all are seen together, they form a white light. "The whole is much greater than the sum of the parts." When all aspects of ourselves are in harmony, we are whole. There are seven aspects that make up the whole person.

Our Inner Self is the central unchanging core of our being, a source of strength and comfort. It relates to the world around us through the physical body, the intellect, the emotions, and the subconscious; to the earth and the cosmos through the energy body; and to the universal mind through the higher self.

Our Higher Self provides us with a meaning in life, with ethical and moral values, and with the highest form of love and compassion.

Our Intellect enables us to communicate with others, to analyze, and to think logically.

Our Subconscious coordinates the functions of our body, our defenses against external threats, and our self-healing, and stores our memories, beliefs, fears, and complexes. It can be programmed for health or for ill health by us, whether consciously or unconsciously.

Our Emotions help us to relate to people and events, and largely determine whether our attitude to life will be positive or negative.

Our Energy Body provides a blueprint for our physical body. We are "beings of energy in a sea of energy." Nothing can manifest in the physical world unless there is some form of energy associated with it. Professor Burr of Yale was the first Westerner to suggest that each of us has an energy body. What he said, in essence, is that disease manifests on the energy body before it shows as symptoms on the physical body.

The energy body is charged partly with electromagnetism and partly with life energy. These are taken in from food, water, air, and light, the latter being just as important to us as it is to plants.

Our Physical Body links us to the physical world to manifest our destiny on earth. If any aspect of ourselves is out of harmony, this will appear as a symptom of the body, as pain or discomfort of some kind.

Outside of our human model, there is the Universal Mind, which has been given many names—Collective Consciousness, Nature, God, Jehovah, The Creator. Through our higher self, we can make contact with the Universal Mind, thus receiving help and guidance and strength to develop ourselves as whole beings.

We are dependent, as well, on our environment for the quality of our life, the light that surrounds us, for the food we eat, the air we breathe, the water we drink, and the energy fields which sustain us.

To become a whole and healthy being, all of our windows must be fully open and interconnected and balanced. When they are, we will be in harmony within ourselves and with our environment.

COMMUNICATION AND RELATIONSHIPS

We spoke at the beginning of this chapter about the need for community situations where the human touch would be normal in all relationships. The single greatest difficulty to overcome in relationships is that of *communication* between individuals. This problem exists everywhere that individuals interact.

The results of lack of communication in the health services are obvious. In the United States, dissatisfied patients are involved in litigation for enormous sums of money because of unnecessary or unsuccessful operations or treatment. Where good rapport has been established between the doctor and the patient, these court cases are minimized. In the United Kingdom, the Health Service is in disarray because of lack of communication at all levels, and this results in strikes and go-slows. The doctor-patient relationship is at an all-time low largely because the average general practitioner can only devote five to six minutes to each patient. What sort of rapport can be established in that time? Time is clearly of the essence in good communication.

Good relationships require communication on all levels, a condition very difficult to achieve in a society where the practitioner has been carefully trained not to become involved with patients on the emotional level, and where the teacher may feel that her only necessary contact with the pupil is on the intellectual level. Mothers may train their children to avoid bodily contact with others who might be unclean. The list can go on and on.

Figure 2 shows an idealized relationship pattern in which we can live and work with others and develop our full potential. When we work in this kind of harmony, extra energy and inspiration enter the relationships.

The diagram shows two individuals, perhaps a mother and child, or a doctor and patient, or teacher and pupil. Each has the potential to be a whole being and to communicate with the other person through all the windows shown.

The closest relationship which can exist is that of mother and child. They are one when the child is in the womb and their central nervous systems are linked. When the child is born and begins to grow, each aspect of his character develops. Finally, there is a need to achieve independence, but a strong link will still exist between the two.

The inner self communicates via the energy body by means of radiations of different forms, difficult to understand or describe, but nonetheless real. The physical body communicates in many ways. Breast-feeding, kissing, and caressing are ways in which a mother conveys sensations to the child. The touch of a loving mother is a wonderful help in healing the child's small hurts. The mother's touching and kissing and hand-holding all help to build a sense of security and a feeling of being needed in the growing child.

All of the other senses—taste, smell, and eye-contact—enter into the parent-child relationship in many ways.

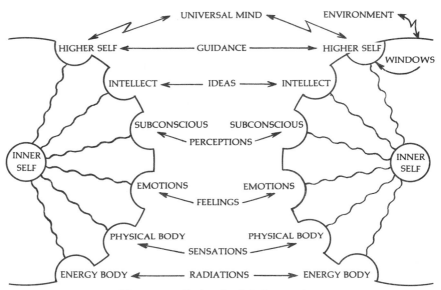

Figure 2. Individual Relationships

A wide spectrum of feelings is generated between a mother and child. The mother may radiate love, serenity, calmness, and confidence, and the child tuning in to these vibrations will undoubtedly respond happily. If the mother is continually upset, under great stress and tension, or radiating lack of interest, fear, worry, hate, anxiety, guilt, or other negative emotions, the child will very likely feel insecure and be difficult, nervous, and full of allergies; the growth pattern may well be stunted.

On the subconscious level, there may well be a link between mother and child manifested in the form of extrasensory perception, as intuition or even telepathy.

At the intellectual level, there is an exchange of ideas between the parent and the child. The relationship is a constantly changing one, and this requires understanding on the part of the mother as the child begins to develop an intellect that requires stimulation from different sources.

Where the higher self of the mother has been developed, the

child will receive guidance regarding values in life. Where the inner self of the mother relates to that of the child at all levels, the much-loved child returns love, and a deep and lasting relationship will build up between the two.

THE DOCTOR-PATIENT RELATIONSHIP

Since we are thinking about health care by considering human relationships, let us go back now to the doctor-patient relationship. Between a mother and child, we have said, love, time, continuity, and a holistic approach are important. All of these are equally important in a doctor-patient relationship. To achieve this, great changes in attitudes and training methods will be required. Let us see what could be achieved.

The effect of the energy body of the doctor on the patient is not really understood at this time, nor is therapeutic touch (or healing) generally accepted by the medical profession.

On the level of the physical body, many modern doctors do not realize the importance of, or shy away from, personal contact with the patient. It is common practice to place a desk or table between the doctor and the patient, and to invite a third person into the clinic during physical examinations. As far as emotions are concerned, medical students are deliberately taught to be objective and not to become emotionally involved with patients. Thus, the patient is kept at a safe distance. There often is little time for the interview and no time at all to build a close rapport between patient and doctor. If the doctor could feel free to put an arm around a patient and encourage him or her to cry, to release built-up tension, it would help to build up the necessary rapport. The truth is that, in many cases, the doctor himself is the best therapy available, but he is so hampered by professional restrictions that his natural abilities are stifled.

Because their teaching is so specifically "scientific," students are taught little or nothing about perception at the nonphysical level. And yet many doctors, nurses, and other health professionals use intuition and other extrasensory faculties in their work, whether consciously or unconsciously! The importance of reintroducing these faculties and making them respectable cannot be overstressed. They are not difficult to develop and are extremely useful as a method of building good relationships between two people.

A doctor can only help a patient to the limit of his own understanding. If the doctor has not developed himself as a whole being and does not have an active higher self, he will be unable to help the patient who is seeking a healthy balance in his life. He will also have a difficult time dealing with the concept of death, and his inability to talk with his patient about it will cause unnecessary tension and distress for both of them.

It is clearly necessary to move ahead with the study of relationships and communication between individuals in the health field and to make the human touch and the emphasis on the individual person accepted in whatever health care plans we develop.

POSITIVE HEALTH

We spoke at the beginning of this chapter of the coming shift to a low-cost system where the main emphasis is on the promotion of health and the secondary emphasis on the cure of illness.

It seems appropriate at this time to think about positive health and to decide what we mean by this term. The idea of positive health is little understood by the general public, and health education, when it exists at all, is so dull and uninteresting to the average child that the whole subject is in the doldrums. We obviously need a new approach.

A simple diagram can help us to understand that positive health is a way of life—a way of thinking and behaving. It brings fulfillment and happiness, and it is catching. It involves working in harmony with nature, and it is exciting and fun. It is based on these simple ideas (Figure 3).

It is important to note that health is not seen as something passive. It becomes an activity, where each action impinges on and affects every other, and ultimately helps us to achieve and maintain health and wholeness.

Only when we have a purpose in life does everything we do have meaning, excitement, and direction. When we think and act positively, we attract to us others who are in tune with us, and wonderful things begin to happen. When we seek to develop the remarkable hidden abilities we all possess, we can use them to help ourselves and others.

Our will is at the center of our being. When we develop the will to be whole and healthy, our life and our health begin to change.

As we learn to adapt to the people and conditions around us, we begin to work in harmony with nature. When we learn to cooperate with and help others, we find that we are giving and receiving love and friendship. When we accept responsibility for our own thoughts and actions, we develop a feeling of freedom and fulfillment, and we know that we can be masters of our own fate.

Finally, what model can we suggest to incorporate the conflicting requirements of cost and time, of relationships and the human touch, of decentralization and individual and community responsibility? How best can we deal with the shift from a "repair" to a "health" philosophy and bring about the integration of all forms of diagnosis and therapy, old and new? How best can we bring about the development and use of people's hidden abilities and how can we most successfully deploy the resources of manpower, money, and equipment which are at present available in the health-care system? The changes are going to be dramatic and far-reaching.

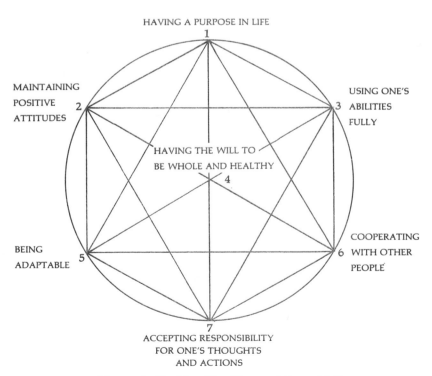

Figure 3. Positive Health as a Way of Life

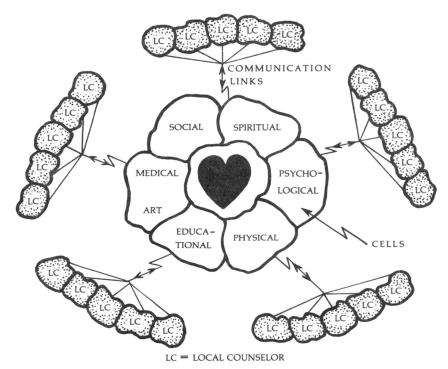

LC = LOCAL COUNSELOR

Figure 4. Model for a Caring Community

A possible model is described here in Figure 4.

The underlying principles involved in this model are, first, that respect for the individual is more important than any consideration of race, creed, nationality, personal status, or scientific investigation; and, second, that pain and suffering call for help based upon compassion, love, sympathy, and sensitivity. It is also assumed that we all have the potential to become whole and healthy beings, but that we may require help at every level of our being to achieve a true balance of spiritual and material values.

The priorities of the system will be: promotion of positive health; prevention of avoidable illness; cure of unavoidable illness; and rehabilitation. Counseling and advice will be provided by individuals who have time to listen to problems—to provide positive health education, and to show how problems and ill health can offer a challenge and provide lessons for the future.

Integration of all forms of diagnosis and therapy will ensure greater simplicity of operation and lower costs. Decentralization to the community and to individuals, together with the responsibility and authority to act where there is need, will help everyone involved with health care to develop his abilities, and delays will be reduced to a minimum. Individuals, families, and the community will be responsible for their own thoughts, actions, health, and quality of life. Continuing relationships, understanding, and trust among everyone in the community and between the community and those who seek help will provide the basis for a happy, holistic community.

In each geographically defined area containing ten or fifteen thousand people, it is expected that a community spirit will grow until the need is felt to manifest, through small groups of individuals, small cells where those who have problems of different types can find advice and help. Gradually, these cells will grow together to form the model described, or something similar to it. This is not a blueprint; each community will see the need somewhat differently.

A caring community would have at its center a heart and a soul around which cells can grow organically to meet needs as they arise while individuals are being treated as whole beings. Typical cells which could be expected to grow are:

Social—a warm and friendly place where young and old can meet, talk, make friends, and develop the community spirit.

Spiritual—one or more beautiful rooms where counsel and help can be given regarding spiritual matters; where healing can be given and received; where meditation groups can meet; where the atmosphere would be one of love and sharing; and a place where old as well as young can find fulfillment.

Psychological—a place where advice and help would be available from qualified counselors who have time to discuss mental and emotional problems, and who work with love, understanding and sensitivity.

Physical—a place dedicated to the development and physical well-being of the body, a place for relaxation, exercise, and fun. Yoga would be taught as well as gymnastics, massage, dancing, rhythm, posture, music, and all aspects of good nutrition.

Educational—cells that would grow in educational establishments, in industry, in the home, or anywhere that a few individuals wish to gather together to learn. Doctors and local counselors would be responsible for instruction using the latest teaching methods.

Medical Art—cells devoted to the practice of an integrated system of conventional and unconventional diagnosis and treatment designed to locate and remove the underlying causes of health problems, and to provide whatever is needed by those who come for help, whether it be acupuncture or drugs, dentistry or diet, medical help or spiritual healing.

The Local Counselors indicated on the diagram are part of a health care system which provides self-help in the home, advice and help as needed by the local counselor, services available in the different cells described, and, when needed, the area hospital.

It has been seen that many problems manifesting as illness can be dealt with by nondoctors. Perhaps 15 percent of such problems really need the doctor and 5 percent the hospital.

The local counselors would need to be warm, mature, comfortable persons who would have time to listen to problems and discuss them with sensitivity for the feelings of the client. They would have responsibility to act in cases of need. They would work as part of a team of five or six counselors and one general practitioner. These counselors could be recruited from a variety of existing grades of health professionals including nurses and social workers, and they could be assisted by lay helpers. Each team would be responsible for a geographical area containing approximately four hundred souls.

This book is about holistic health. It refers frequently to the unity of body, mind and spirit which is the foundation of holism. In this chapter, we have ventured to look into the future and to describe what the feelings, attitudes, and relationships must be before we can establish a new model for health care. What we are describing may seem idealistic and utopian. Perhaps it is—but if the new model is undergirded with sound principles, then there is no reason why it cannot eventually grow as we have visualized it.

35

The Longest Stride of Soul Man Ever Took

EILEEN NOAKES

Who can doubt that the world is undergoing some major upheaval, with war, strikes, oppression, and murder so common as to be commonplace? And yet, there is an unreasonable exhilaration, a feeling of preparation for a great leap forward. We seem to be aware of a great inner energy shaping events. I want to suggest the paradox that, despite the turmoil, on the one hand "not a grain of sand is out of place" and "the everlasting arms are underneath"; yet, on the other, *our* efforts, individual and collective, are essential to the emergence from this crisis of the kind of world we dream of for ourselves, our children and our grandchildren.

There is a Divine plan which underlies the manifested world, but it can only emerge as its various aspects find centers of reception in us. No astute political formulas, no clever economic juggling, will provide the answer, for it lies within us. Many people, of course, long only for a return to stability, order, security, and personal comfort, but this will no longer do. A *new* world is being unveiled, and much new energy is pouring into the planet, but, while the blueprint exists, the building is our task. It is wise to cooperate with the forces of change so that we shall not be swept along and possibly submerged by the tidal wave of irresistible energy. We are here at this time for a purpose. We have elected to incarnate at what must be one of the most dramatic and challenging periods in the history of the planet, and we must not miss the opportunity to play our destined part.

This might be called a crisis of consciousness. Richard Bucke postulates the theory of a gradual evolution of consciousness,

punctuated by periodic giant leaps, such as those which characterized the birth of simple and self consciousness. We are now,
he believes, engaged in another giant leap—into Cosmic Consciousness.[1]

This coming civilization, we are assured, carries the promise of
beauty, love, creativity, and brotherhood beyond our wildest
imaginings, but we need to stand firm, strongly centered between
the Earthly Mother and the Heavenly Father. *We* are the mediators
between the inner and outer worlds, and it is our task to anchor
these energies and express them in form, both by constructive
thinking and planning on every level—community, national,
worldwide—and, as Alice A. Bailey says in *Rays and Initiations*,[2] by
"demonstrating in our environment the qualities which will establish right human relations and show on a small scale the behavior which will some day characterize enlightened humanity."

THE AGE OF THE GROUP IMPULSE

The Aquarian Age is the age of the group impulse, of the stimulation of cooperation and group endeavor in the place of competition and personal ambition. Yet, we need to recognize that the
negative application of this energy could lead to totalitarianism
and the crushing of individuality. In response to this impulse,
many groups have begun to form, both on inner levels and on
outer physical levels. Many feel an urgent need to express this
impulse in a creative, constructive life-style which will vibrate in
tune with the higher energies and bring healing to humanity and
the planet, for wholeness is to be found not in the curing of
symptoms, but in the practice of holistic living.

A group of people living, working and meditating together can
generate power which is greater than the sum total of their individual energy. This might take the form of a return to village life,
but a return on a higher turn of the spiral, with a conscious feeling
of community and a commitment to the expression of the spiritual
on every level and in every activity.

So, much of the responsibility for ushering in the New Age is
ours, and we need to provide efficient vehicles for the work that
has to be done. We are sparks of Divine life, individualizing
through souls which inhabit a threefold personality, the physi-
cal/etheric body, the astral or emotional body, and the mental

body; all these levels need to be active, developed, and aligned for the task ahead.

THE PHYSICAL BODY

First of all, the physical body merits our care and respect both as a gift from the Earthly Mother and as the Temple of the Spirit. The Ageless Wisdom and the Essenes suggest that it is impossible for higher knowledge and guidance to be transmitted through a coarse physical body, and we are given clear and practical advice for its refinement.

We have a fundamental need to be in touch with the rhythms and cycles of nature. One way of answering this need is to be in close touch with the soil by growing our own vegetables organically and being relatively self-sufficient. This puts us more in charge of our own lives, provides us with living, unadulterated food, and makes a contribution to the world food supply. Diet is an important factor in our well-being, and many people are beginning to accept that the healthiest diet consists largely of fruit and raw vegetables—living food.

The Essenes, whose practice of community living could hardly be improved upon, ate simple meals of uncooked food only twice a day. They also demonstrated that understanding natural laws and living in harmony with natural forces enabled them to produce sufficient food for their needs and a surplus for distribution to the poor in only four hours a day, leaving ample time for other creative activities. We could revolutionize our consumption of food and fuel if we adopted this practice. Shortages are created, at least partly, by our artificial demands and our demands for artificiality. There would be less need for healing from other sources if simplicity were implicit in our life-styles, in a rhythm of good, constructive work, alternating with relaxation and mental and spiritual stimulation, in an atmosphere of caring and concern; the study and application of total physical relaxation; the exploration of the inner world of myth and symbol, and the acceptance of responsibility for our own lives. We also need the opportunity to develop creative skills and talents and to express ourselves through drama and dance.

I don't believe that the true cause of inflation and the proliferation of strikes is material need. I feel that people are really trying to express the frustration of uncreative work, lack of involvement, and unbalanced, stultified life-styles; but nobody in public life seems to challenge the underlying assumption that an ever-spiraling standard of living is a life-enhancing goal. Certainly, basic needs must be met before the higher satisfactions can be enjoyed, but they are not in themselves a source of fulfillment.

THE ASTRAL BODY

A very large proportion of ill-health has its origin in the astral or emotional body. A free flow of energy is vital from the astral body to the physical/etheric, through the chakras to the endocrine glands, and thence to the organs of the body; but many blockages are caused by the destructive emotions, and especially by suppressed emotion and the rejection of pain. Our emotional health depends on taking responsibility for our own lives and accepting every situation, every contact, every relationship, as expressly designed by the soul to stimulate growth and the removal of blockages. Every rejected experience is pushed down into the subconscious, creating a vacuum into which is sucked an exact reflection of that energy. The outer world reflects with uncanny accuracy our inner projections, and there is no one we can, or have any right to, change except ourselves. All is God, and we are surrounded by and moving through those aspects of God that we have drawn to ourselves, like magnets creating a pattern with iron filings. It's not easy to see the Face of God in the plight of starving children, homeless refugees, and oppressed peoples except by recognizing that, on a different level of truth and reality, these sufferings have both dignity and meaning, and cease to be. Just beyond our vision, the world is shining with love, and, if we see this truth and hold firmly to it, we shall help to dissolve the veils that enshroud us in the world of form and matter. This is not at all the same as saying that we should view these things with complacency or fail to do everything we can to alleviate distress.

LOVE—THE GLUE OF THE UNIVERSE

In our search for the key to the good life, we keep coming back to the word *love*, which seems to be the glue of the Universe, a reflection in quantum physics of the particle "charm" which holds everything together. If we live in love, we live in harmony; if we hate, we harm everything we touch, but mostly ourselves. Our emotions do not evaporate without trace; they coalesce with other similar emotions to form clouds of anger, hatred, or joy, which we both expand and attract to us, so that a mood of irritation can quickly and unaccountably escalate into uncontrollable rage. On the other hand, love is equally infectious, so that to "love one's neighbor as oneself" was the best psychology and the most practical advice ever given. It is so often mistaken as an injunction to be pious or inoffensive, but, in fact, to love is sheer magic, a dynamic force which is totally irresistible and which can transform any situation. It packs tremendous power, not in an abstract way, or on some far-distant level, but here and now and literally. Projecting love is as real as watering plants with fertilizer, and much more potent, because the effect is often instantaneous.

I've heard it said that, when you're in love, the air seems a remarkable medium to be moving through, but the fact is that we *are* "In Love" in capital letters, and it *is* a remarkable medium to be moving through. Awareness of this marks the point in our evolution when frustration, loneliness, and pain begin to be replaced by joy, which is not the same as happiness, because joy is independent of circumstances.

It is said that, during the course of our lives from conception to the grave, we recapitulate the stages of evolution. We develop, in the same order as the race, faculties such as memory, simple consciousness, remorse, self-consciousness, a moral nature, and so on. For his protection, primitive man was equipped with a "flight or fight" response. At the onset of anger or fear, the midbrain sends a message to the organs of the body to prepare for action. This stage of being, motivated by self-preservation and self-defense, corresponds with simple consciousness in the race and the age of up to three years in a child, but many of us have not developed beyond this stage. Unconsciously, our reactions are still automatically triggered by a search for security or sensation, and, since these are needs which can never be satisfied, we spend our lives in a frenzied pursuit of the unattainable. We may have become skillful at concealing it by sophisticated rationalization, but basically we still twitch at imaginary threats to our survival. Having served us extremely well in the past, the old programming needs to be replaced by something quite different. Our future survival depends on good will in place of defensiveness and self-interest, and this is an urgent need, not a pious hope.

THE BIRTH OF SELF-CONSCIOUSNESS

The next great leap in consciousness in the race was the birth of self-consciousness, when man for the first time was able to stand outside of himself and observe himself, when he was no longer totally immersed in his sensations. This is achieved at something like three years in a child. It is characterized by self-centeredness rather than instinct, by self-expression, aggrandizement, competitiveness. Having achieved the basic necessities, the next search is for love, but, even here, we may continue to apply jungle techniques. Our love is conditional, it is possessive, it makes demands. It is, in fact, simply loving a part of ourselves projected onto another. We are beginning to question the value of marriage as an institution, but I don't think that marriage has necessarily failed. I believe the failure lies in unresolved repressions finding mirror images. Marriage does not need to be a prison; it can be a union of two mature beings standing side by side, contributing to each other's growth. At its highest level, it reflects a great cosmic truth, the balancing of polarities, the union of opposites, but it can be expressed on any level, right down to the most primitive. Instead of recognizing that the level we have chosen reflects an aspect of our own development, we look for reasons of failure in outward circumstances. Mostly, we are attracted to somebody who either mirrors a repressed conflict or who supplies our inadequacies. Only the mature can expect a mature relationship, because it takes maturity to love, not just to be in love. One of the most liberating experiences in the world is the decision to love unconditionally, not to feel the need to reform people, nor to take offense.

Practicing love also means practicing "harmlessness," which, although it requires that our thoughts, words and deeds be harmless, is not negative or mere abstention from evil, but a very positive applicaton of good will. It may require firmness and the ability to say no, but it will be compassionate and uncritical, though not necessarily lacking in discrimination. It will not be sentimental, and it will not be weak for the sake of popularity or peace. It will not be possessive and it will not demand ego fulfilment. The practice of love is an excellent method of clearing clogged channels so that higher energies can flow in.

Blockages in the emotional body can be compared to cholesterol in the arteries of the physical body, and many techniques have been developed to help us "clear the channels." To touch briefly on a few:

1. The use of physical relaxation to help break the pattern of response to anger or fear by the ancient "flight or fight" mechanism.
2. The use of the "evening review," which is a survey of the day's actions and reactions last thing at night from the angle of an objective observer, apportioning neither praise nor blame, but simply noting dispassionately. It is thought that this acts as a clearing process and frees our dreams for more creative work.
3. The use of the creative imagination—
    a. By making the morning resolve—tuning into the day's program and seeing it directed by one's higher self.
    b. By contacting one's inner guide, using such methods as transpersonal psychology, guided daydreams, or meditations.

We so often believe ourselves to be alone. Never for one moment is this true. It's an illusion contained in our descent into matter, but we are now ⊂ ι the evolutionary arc, and the veil between the visible and invis.ble is beginning to dissolve. "The Elder Brothers of the race who have guided humanity through the long centuries are now preparing people for the next great step. This step will bring in a continuity of consciousness which will do away with the fear of death, and link the physical and astral planes in such close relationship that they will in reality constitute one plane."[3]

PROGRESS TO HIGHER CONSCIOUSNESS

It takes a long time for a development in consciousness to be attained by the whole human race. Some people are still moving from simple to self-consciousness, but, gradually, idealistic man is emerging, the world server, detached from personal interests, cooperative, unpossessive, wishing to understand the plan of creation and to serve God. Certainly there are people who have attained some degree at least of the higher or intuitional consciousness. The descriptions of moments of illumination tally remarkably. They use terms like apprehensions of beauty, unity, light, love—but, above all, unity, all of us members one of another in a universe filled with love. This is what I believe Martin Luther King experienced when he said, "God has led me to the top of the mountain, and I have looked over the other side. Mine eyes have seen the glory of the coming of the Lord. I no longer have fear."

This is what lies ahead of us, just a blink away. But again, here is the paradox. Yes, it's coming, we're experiencing the birth pangs of a New Age with a higher consciousness, but it is our responsibility to usher it in, through our meditations and the quality of our loving.

Having developed the intellect, we then need to silence it to develop this higher form of knowing, using the creative imagination to build the Rainbow Bridge firstly between the little self and the soul, and then between the soul and the spirit, where guidance and inspiration are to be found which then need to be translated into action in a very practical and efficient way.

We will eventually discover that, after we have made this "longest stride of soul," the New Age will come, not as a result of reaching upward or straining outward, but of seeing what was there all the time!

An End—and a Beginning

I n this book, we have been on a journey toward wholeness. When we started out, we knew it would be a voyage of discovery, but we were not entirely sure what kind of an experience it would be. It is rather like looking at a map before you go off on a trip and saying, "Oh, I've always wanted to go there!" and "We really *must* spend a few days here—it's supposed to be fabulous!" In real life, there are sometimes disappointments and always surprises. The fabulous spot is overcrowded and overrated, and perhaps some little, unheard-of place proves much more rewarding.

No travel agent could have described the journey we have just taken or prepared us for the adventures along the way. We started out with our usual enthusiasm for travel, and with the conviction that it was going to be challenging and fun and that, whatever happened along the way, we would return with new friends and new insights, and a collection of wonderful new pictures for our mind galleries!

We have crossed boundaries and time lines, traveled to high places where the going was sometimes difficult, occasionally lost our way for a bit, and then found the track again.

Many times we saw signs that tempted us to explore in different directions. But we knew that, despite our desire for adventure and excitement, we *did* have a goal ahead. Our journey, and yours, as you followed us, has been toward a holistic way of living, toward the wholeness of the individual person who seeks a path to follow.

Now we are all together on the journey to greater understanding. You, the reader, have become a part of us, the editors and contributors. We now share a common language and have some perceptions in common. One of those perceptions is that, whenever our trip takes us to the answer to one question, we look up to find three or four more questions staring us in the face! But this is not discouraging; it is part of the fun and the challenge. It's just like climbing to the crest of a hill to discover a dazzling view and then seeing another hill to yet another exciting view waiting.

No journey begins at one point and stops at another. Every journey begins long before you climb onto the train, and ends only by becoming the beginning of another adventure. We hope that reaching the end of this book is a real beginning for you— that it has taken you to places you always hoped to visit—and that it has answered a few questions about holistic health, and about the unity of body, mind, and spirit!

PETER AND BETS ALBRIGHT

About the Authors

Having gone on this journey towards wholeness, you will certainly wish to be acquainted with those who have helped to make the journey exciting. All of the contributors to this book are listed below in alphabetical order.

Bets Parker Albright Bets Albright was born in Franconia, New Hampshire, but grew up in New York City where she attended an assortment of private schools as well as the King–Coit Childrens' Theatre. She was graduated from Wellesley College. In 1953, she and her husband, Scudder M. Parker, left Westchester County, New York, and moved to High Reach Farm in North Danville, Vermont. In 1957, after their house was destroyed by fire, Bets and her husband and five children spent several years in Hardwick and Newport, Vermont, where Scudder served as minister to several small churches. After Scudder Parker's death in 1966, Bets returned to High Reach Farm, and, in 1968, she married Peter Albright. The Albrights live at the North Danville farm. Bets writes stories for children and is actively involved in many aspects of holistic health, including nutrition, herbs, and reflexology. She is a staff associate at Pathways to Well-Being, a center for holistic health in Burlington, Vermont. She has been a dowser for some years and is a trustee of the American Society of Dowsers, which has its headquarters in Danville, Vermont.

Peter Albright Peter Albright has been a resident of the northeastern United States nearly all his life and of Vermont since 1963. He studied orthodox medicine at Allegheny College, Pennsylvania (B.A., 1949) and Cornell University Medical College (M.D., 1953). His residency training in internal medicine was at Cleveland Clinic in Ohio (1954–1957). He practiced orthodox medicine from 1957 to 1976, and his special interests included nutrition, geriatrics, rehabilitation, and environmental health. In 1978–79, he was

295

president of the Vermont State Medical Society. His interest in alternatives in health began in the early 1970s, and he has studied various aspects of healing in the United States and Britain since that time. He has been actively involved in the development of a holistic health center in northern Vermont. Peter is now practicing holistic medicine at Pathways to Well-Being, a center for holistic health in Burlington, Vermont. He belongs to the American Holistic Medical Association, the Vermont State Medical Society, the Scientific and Medical Network (Great Britain), The American Society of Dowsers, and the International Biogenic Society.

Anne Oliver Bassage   Anne Bassage has been a Vermonter since she was twelve years old. Her farm, Fifer's Ride, in East Calais, is the embodiment of all the old houses she used to see and dream of remodeling in Vermont. She graduated from Vassar College in 1935 and taught zoology there for three years. She has been interested in holistic health since she learned that she is a hypoglycemic and has been able to halt her distressing symptoms by vitamin and mineral therapy, and diet. Her high blood pressure caused her to seek biofeedback learning which she did with Ruth McCollester of Greenwich, Connecticut. Anne now practices during the summer in East Calais, and in the winter in Darien, Connecticut. She has done workshops for the Vermont Mental Health Association, the University of Vermont, Vermont College and private groups. She appeared with Jack Barry on Vermont Educational Television in a half hour demonstration of biofeedback. Her most recent study has been with Dr. Elmer Green, his wife Alyce, and their research team at the Menninger Foundation in Topeka, Kansas. She is a member of the Biofeedback Society of America.

Devaki Berkson   Born in Chicago, Devaki Berkson is a graduate of the University of Michigan. Several years ago, because of a painful and disabling illness which resisted medical and even surgical treatment, she began treatment at the hands of a foot reflexologist. Her diet was reformed, and she started a specific exercise program. Soon, her problems abated entirely. This experience led her to study health on all levels. She received a master's degree in nutrition from Goddard College. She is a certified shiatsu therapist and has lectured and taught at numerous yoga centers. She also studied foot reflexology extensively, and, in 1977, she wrote *The Foot Book*. She received the degree of Doctor of Chiropractic in 1979 from Western States Chiropractic College. Through prolonged and intensive study, Devaki has made herself an authority on a broad range of closely allied approaches to health and has become a model for other holistic practitioners to follow.

Anne Coulter Anne Coulter was born in Minnesota, but spent summers as a child in an old Vermont farmhouse and vowed to return one day. She did so and has lived in Vermont for eight years. She is a graduate of Brown University and has worked for a newspaper, Vista, and the American Friends Service Committee. She worked for a time at a community medical clinic in Baltimore, Maryland, and now divides her time between the St. Johnsbury office of Planned Parenthood of Vermont and the Danville, Vermont Health Center.

Barbara D'Arcy-Thompson Barbara D'Arcy-Thompson is the daughter of Sir D'Arcy-Thompson, formerly Professor of Natural History at St. Andrews University in Scotland and author of the classic work *On Growth and Form*. Barbara, now retired from academic life, lives at the Findhorn Foundation in Forres, Scotland. Her greatest interest lies in healing and wholeness. She has studied massage, reflexology and prenatal therapy in depth, and practices with an intuitive understanding of the underlying causes of imbalance. She has visited the United States several times and has given workshops in reflexology and prenatal therapy while here.

Adele Dawson Adele Dawson is a geographical transplant, but Marshfield, Vermont has been her home for twenty years. Her herb and vegetable gardens wander up a forty-five degree hill overlooking a waterfall. Herbalist, painter, woodcarver, teacher and lecturer, she calls these occupations creative transformation. Adele is an active member of the Herb Society of Vermont and an enthusiastic student and supporter of holistic health. Her book, *Health, Happiness, and the Pursuit of Herbs*, is published by The Stephen Greene Press.

Marc Estrin Marc Estrin is enjoying a unique career blending the healing and performing arts. He was elected to Phi Beta Kappa in his junior year and graduated from Queens College in New York with highest honors, concentrating in music, chemistry and biology. He then had a two-year fellowship at Rockefeller Institute in microbiology, following which he earned a Master's Degree in theater arts at the University of California at Los Angeles. Marc produced, directed and taught in a number of theatre projects in different parts of the U.S. over the next six years. Ten years ago, he became a faculty member at Goddard College in Vermont, a position which he held until two years ago, teaching various subjects, including music, theater, science, politics, and philosophy. Five years ago, he enrolled in a program which led to his becoming a certified physician's assistant, and he has also become a certified emergency medical technician. He has made an independent study of oriental medicine and uses shiatsu as a part of his clinical practice. He is currently working as a physician's assistant in a holistic health center in northern Vermont.

Edward P. Jastram   Edward Jastram is a native of Providence, Rhode Island, now living in Rehoboth, Massachusetts. He graduated from M.I.T. in 1935, majoring in physics. He followed an industrial career with Metals and Controls Corporation of Attleboro, Massachusetts, which merged with Texas Instruments, Inc. in 1958. He was variously chief engineer, manager of research and manager of advanced planning. He retired in 1974. He began dowsing in 1954. It developed rapidly for him as a method of general problem solving, appearing to be a method of ESP, a part of general psychic functioning. He is both a member and a trustee of the American Society of Dowsers. He also belongs to the British Society of Dowsers, The American Society for Psychical Research, The Parapsychology Foundation, Inc., and the Huna Research Associates.

Donald R. Land   Donald Land is founder and director of Nutrition Information Systems, a privately operated information agency providing foodservice consulting and nutrition education services to institutions. His professional activities have included being Assistant Professor of Computer Science, Assistant Professor of Chemistry, food and nutrition instructor, research analytical chemist, computer programmer analyst, systems analyst and co-founder of an alternative experimental college. He has also had extensive public experience, including being Commissioner for the New Hampshire State Human Rights Commission, the organization of minority and low–income communities, and founder and director of a volunteer community–action program. As director of N.I.S. since 1976, he has developed a clientele throughout New England that includes Head Start centers, day–care centers, schools, camps, juvenile homes, mental health agencies, gerontology agencies, private and professional agencies and human service agencies. He received degrees in chemistry from U.C.L.A. (Ph.D), Howard University and the University of New Hampshire. Born in Portland, Oregon in 1935, he grew up in Los Angeles, he studied in Washington, D.C. and moved to Durham, N.H. in 1964, where he now resides.

Marcus McCausland   Marcus McCausland and his wife, Marika, are responsible for the formation of the foundation known as Health for the New Age in England in 1972. After studying law at Cambridge, Marcus served for 29 years in the regular Army, retiring as Lieutenant Colonel. He then spent five years in the electronics industry, which he considers to be good preparation for his life's work: establishing a network of friends and contacts throughout the world among members of the medical profession, scientists, ministers of religion, unconventional therapists and the general public. For ten years, he has studied health, ill health, relationships, the integration of different methods of diagnosis and therapy, nutrition, health education, and the changes taking place in western medicine. He is responsible for the publication of a quarterly newsletter, *Trends in Health Care,* and for a treatise, *Nutrition Research: The Need for an Innovative Approach.*

Oscar L. Morphis   Oscar Morphis has worked for many years as a cancer specialist in Fort Worth, Texas. For the past several years, he has worked in partnership with Dr. Carl Simonton, whose work with visual imagery in cancer therapy is known world–wide. He received his M.D. degree from Southwestern Medical School of the University of Texas. Dr. Morphis is a fellow of the American College of Radiology, the Society of Clinical and Experimental Hypnosis, the Academy of Psychosomatic Medicine, the International Academy of Preventive Medicine and the American College of Nuclear Medicine. Through intensive study, he has developed a deep understanding of modern physics and has become an authority in the field of human energy and energy transfer systems as they relate to health, sickness and healing. He has lectured extensively throughout the U.S. on these and other subjects.

Eileen Noakes   Eileen Noakes, a native of South Africa, has run a healing center in Devon, England for many years where she has done spiritual teaching, massage, deep relaxation therapy, counseling and healing. She hopes very much to establish in Devon an Essene community which will incorporate a healing center. Eileen was a founder of the Scientific and Medical Network in Britain, and she is a trustee of the Human Development Trust. She is in great demand as a lecturer and has spoken numerous times at Findhorn in Scotland and at Paul Solomon's Fellowship of the Inner Light at Virginia Beach.

John Nutting   John Nutting came to Vermont in 1956 from Duluth, Minnesota, where he was born and raised. He served as pastor of the Congregational churches in Hyde Park and North Hyde Park for ten years. Since that time, he has been a member of the staff of the Vermont Conference of the United Church of Christ. He has spent much of his time working with low-income and other disadvantaged people in Vermont's many small villages. He learned to play the guitar, composed over 100 songs, and made a record, *Songs of Lamoille County*. He is married to Ramona Russell and lives in Shutesville.

Scudder H. Parker   Scudder Parker is a minister in East St. Johnsbury and Lower Waterford, Vermont. He has combined his ministry in these churches over the past eleven years with working to end the Vietnam war, to reduce military spending, and to get recycling started in northeastern Vermont. He is an authorized teacher of reevaluation counseling, a poet, an enthusiastic dancer and a zealous softball and volleyball player. He is the father of two daughters, Katie, 9 and Emily, 4; and the husband of Pamela, who is a Learning Disabilities Consultant for the Caledonia North Supervisory Union. Scudder is a graduate of Union Theological Seminary in New York City; Williams College, Williamstown, Massachusetts; and Hardwick Academy, Hardwick, Vermont.

Stephen M. Parker   Stephen Parker lives in Danville, Vermont and is a carpenter, part-time farmer and group process trainer. He is a graduate of Williams College. For three years, he lived in the Life Center, a communal situation in Philadelphia, and worked with the Movement for a New Society, a network of social change groups. He has been a teacher of reevaluation counseling for four years and has taught at Goddard College in Plainfield, Vermont.

T. Edward Ross II   Terry Ross is three-term President of the American Society of Dowsers. He is a retired Philadelphia stock-broker, dowser, and researcher in the world of PSI. He says that he became attracted to this field when, as a boy of 11, he watched a Vermonter search for water with a wild apple branch. He feels that the areas of PSI are aspects of the same force, which includes life-after-life, nature spirits, earth forces and healing. He has spo-ken in the U.S. and Britain to groups interested in these subjects. He is convinced that ancient lore is fast becoming modern science and that this will alter the academic scene.

Paul Solomon   Paul Solomon is the son of a minister and has been steeped in the Bible since childhood. He, too, was educated and ordained in the Baptist ministry, but nothing in life had pre-pared him for the mystical experience that launched him, at thirty-three, into a new life, a new ministry, and a new relation-ship with God. His ministry includes clairvoyance, spiritual heal-ing and prophecy, and his use of these abilities in his role as a teacher has won him acclaim as a leader in the Aquarian age. He is the founder of the Fellowship of the Inner Light, which is dedi-cated to uplifting and supporting those entering the realms of spiritual awareness. His students are carefully trained for particu-lar ministries, counseling, teaching and other vocations. Paul has become particularly well-known for his understanding of matters relating to health. He has been able to advise many in this area, using information obtained from his inner source in a manner similar to that of Edgar Cayce. He is much in demand as a speaker and has appeared at many conferences and seminars throughout the U.S., and in Britain, Europe and the Middle East.

Louise Sunfeather   Louise Sunfeather, a graduate of Oberlin College, is the focalizer of Star Seed, an organization working in the community of Burlington, Vermont to explore ways of holistic living. She is a psychotherapist in private practice, an educational and organizational consultant, and a teacher. She has been a human and group relations trainer as well. Her special interest is translating the holistic world view and the behaviors that it generates into our daily lives to support the evolution of our highest potential as individuals and groups.

Patricia Swartz   Patricia Swartz was born and brought up in England. She has taught high school science in England, Switzerland and the U.S. She became a childbirth educator in 1970 and has taught childbirth preparation since then. She was the Vermont coordinator for The American Society for Prophylaxis in Obstetrics for five years, helping to train other childbirth educators and to spread the use of Lamaze childbirth in Vermont and northern New Hampshire. She is employed by Caledonia Home Health Care Agency as a childbirth educator and is a corporator of Northeastern Vermont Regional Hospital. She is married and has three children. Her interests include family and outdoor activities such as gardening, sheep raising, skiing, bicycling, sewing and reading. As a teacher, she is especially interested in fostering consumer awareness.

Susanne Terry   Susanne Terry is a writer and group consultant living in Danville, Vermont. She is a teacher of reevaluation counseling, a peer counseling method that is based on many of the concepts contained in the chapter of this book which she co-authored with Stephen Parker. Her publications include: *Moving Towards a New Society* (New Society Press), and *Building Social Change Communities* (NSP). She was a contributor to *Resource Manual for a Living Revolution* (NSP), and her articles have appeared in *Fellowship Magazine, WIN Magazine, National Catholic Reporter,* and *American Report.*

John F. Thie   John Thie is the director of Thie Chiropractic Corporation in Pasadena and the founding president of the Touch for Health Foundation. He graduated from the University of Southern California and Los Angeles College of Chiropractic (D.C.) and completed postgraduate studies at the University of California at Los Angeles. He is currently a member of the faculty of Pepperdine University of Malibu and the Center for Holistic Studies of Antioch University West, as well as the extension faculties of University of California, Riverside and San Diego, and Los Angeles Valley College. He has made presentations on Touch for Health at the University of California, Berkeley School of Public Health, UCLA's outpatient Pain Control Clinic, the University of Southern California Dental School Acupuncture Study Group, and the Parker Chiropractic Research Foundation. Dr. Thie is a life member of the American Association for the Advancement of Science and is listed in *Leaders of American Science*. He is the founding chairman of the International College of Applied Kinesiology. He has been a faculty member and lecturer at many chiropractic colleges throughout the world. In 1978, traveling with one of the first groups to visit the Peoples Republic of China, he presented Touch for Health to medical personnel in Peking, Shanghai and Nanking. He has served as president of the Los Angeles County Chiropractic Society, has been moderator of the First Congregational Church of Pasadena, and has held numerous civic leadership positions. He lives in Malibu with his wife, Carrie, and their three sons—John Jr., Luther and Matthew—all of whom are active in sharing Touch for Health with the lay public.

Lawrence L. Weed   Lawrence L. Weed is a professor of medicine and community medicine at the University of Vermont College of Medicine. He is well-known throughout the medical and health care professions as the author of a philosophy and system of health care which has been termed the Problem–Oriented System. He now directs the Problem-Oriented Medical Information System (PROMIS) Laboratory, which uses computer technology combined with medical skills in a research effort to develop a more efficient and meaningful patient medical record. Lawrence Weed was educated at Hamilton College in New York (BA, 1943) and Columbia University College of Physicians and Surgeons (MD, 1947). He has worked and studied in many fields in medicine, including biochemistry, microbiology, pharmacology and medical education. Prior to coming to the University of Vermont, he was professor of medicine and director of Out–Patient Clinics of the Cleveland Metropolitan Hospital in Ohio. Dr. Weed believes, and is demonstrating, that holistic care of each patient can be achieved through the computerized Problem-Oriented System, which the patient can use as a tool for coordination and guidance in all encounters with all providers of health care. Dr. Weed has written over forty medical scientific papers, and a book, *Your Health Care and How to Manage It.*

Notes

Introduction   pp. ix–xii

1. Smuts, Jan C. *Holism and Evolution*. New York: Macmillan, 1926.
2. Ibid.

Why People Must Manage Their Own Health Care   pp. 21–35

1. Stravinsky, Igor. *Poetics of Music.* Cambridge, Massachusetts: Harvard University Press, 1942.

Using Inner and Outer Resources   pp. 36–39

1. Shapiro, J., and Shapiro, D. "The Psychology of Responsibility." *New England Journal of Medicine.* 301 (July 26, 1979): 211–212.

The Scientific Method and the Medical Model   pp. 43–52

1. Cade, C. Maxwell, and Coxhead, Nona. *The Awakened Mind.* New York: Delacorte, 1979.
2. Kanellakos, D. P., and Lucas, J. P. *The Psychobiology of Transcendental Meditation.* Menlo Park, California: W. A. Benjamin, 1974.
3. Benson, Herbert. *The Relaxation Response.* New York: Morrow, 1975.
4. Ballantine, Rudolph. *Diet and Nutrition.* Honesdale, Pennsylvania: Himalayan International Institute, 1978.
5. Diamond, John. *Behavioral Kinesiology.* New York: Harper & Row, 1979.
6. McGarey, William A. *Acupuncture and Body Energies.* Phoenix, Arizona: Gabriel Press, 1974.
7. Berkson, Devaki. *The Foot Book.* New York: Funk & Wagnalls, 1977.
8. Dawson, Adele. *Health, Happiness and the Pursuit of Herbs.* Brattleboro, Vermont: Stephen Greene, 1980.
9. American Medical Association. *Principles of Medical Ethics.* Chicago: AMA, 1957.

Cancer: Symbol and Challenge of Our Times   pp. 53–61

1. Szekely, Edmond Bordeaux. *The Essene Way: Biogenic Living.* Costa Rica: International Biogenic Society, 1978.
2. Fisher, Bernard. "Breast Cancer Management: Alternatives to Radical Mastectomy." *New England Journal of Medicine* 301 (August 9, 1979): 326–328.
3. Crile, George, Jr. "Developments in the treatment of cancer of the breast." *Cleveland Clinic Quarterly* 44 (1977): 9–13.
4. Special Report. "Treatment of Primary Breast Cancer." *New England Journal of Medicine* 301 (August 9, 1979): 340.
5. Fisher, op cit., page 327.

Sexuality and Well-Being   pp. 71–80

1. Kinsey, Alfred C., Pomeroy, Wardell and Martin, Clyde E. *Sexual Behavior in the Human Male.* Philadelphia: Saunders, 1948, and Kinsey, Alfred C. *Sexual Behavior in the Human Female.* Philadelphia: Saunders, 1953.

Moving through Life and Dealing with Hurts   pp. 92–101

1. Leboyer, Frederick. *Birth Without Violence.* New York: Knopf, 1975.

Exercise and Yoga: Regaining Our Place of Power   pp. 110–21

1. Katch, F., and McArdle, W. *Nutrition, Weight Control & Exercise.* Boston: Houghton-Mifflin, 1977.
2. Shock, H. in *Scientific American* 206 (1962): 101–110.
3. Raab, W. in *West Virginia Medical Journal* 65 (1969): 1–3.
4. Salzman, S. H., et al. in *Journal of Applied Physiology* 29 (1979): 92–95.
5. *Clinical Trends in Cardiology* 5 (Sept.–Oct. 1975): 7.
6. *Science,* April 7, 1978: 62.
7. *Clinically Speaking* 2 (Jan.–Feb. 1978).
8. Fox, S. M., et al. in *Annals of Clinical Research* 3 (1971): 404–432.
9. Upledger, J. in *Journal of the American Osteopathic Association* 76 (August 1977): 890–896.
10. Retzlaff, —. in *Journal of the American Osteopathic Association* 74 (May 1975): 869–873.
11. Peterson, C. *Digest of Chiropractic Econ.* (March–April 1979): 52.
12. Steer —, and Horney, —. *Canadian Medical Association Journal* 98 (January 13, 1968): 71–74.
13. Fryman, —. *Journal of the American Osteopathic Association* 70 (May 1971): 928–945.

14. Andrew, V. *The Psychic Power of Running*. New York: Rawson, Wade, 1978.
15. Iyengar, B. K. S. *Light on Yoga*. London: Allen and Unwin, 1965.
16. Hall, Felicite. From lecture notes.
17. Kramer, Joel. From lecture notes.
18. *The Lancet* (October 14, 1978): 814.
19. Ott, John. *Health and Light*. New York: Simon and Schuster, 1973.
20. Jensen, Bernard. *You Can Master Disease*. Solara Beach, California: Bernard Jensen Publishing, no date.

Attuning to Our Nourishment   pp. 126–29

1. Szekely, Edmond Bordeaux. *The Essene Way: Biogenic Living*. Costa Rica: International Biogenic Society, 1978.

Food and People: Two Systems Interacting   pp. 130–44

1. Laszlo, E. *The Systems View of the World*. New York: George Braziller, 1972.
2. Ardell, D. *High-level Wellness*. Emmaus, Pennsylvania: Rodale, 1977.
3. Bloomfield, H., and Kory, R. *The Holistic Way to Health and Happiness*. New York: Simon and Schuster, 1978.
4. Williams, R. J., Heffley, J. D., Yew, M., and Bode, C. W. "A Renaissance of Nutritional Science Is Imminent." *Perspectives in Biology and Medicine*, vol. 17, no. 1, 1973.
5. Hall, R. H. *Food for Nought: The Decline In Nutrition*. New York: Vintage, 1976.
6. Williams, *op cit.*
7. Ballentine, R. *Diet and Nutrition*. Himalayan International Institute, 1978.
8. Hall, R. H., *op cit.*
9. Bloomfield, H., *op cit.*
10. Williams, R. J. *Nutrition against Disease*. Toronto: Pitman, 1971.
11. Kalita, D. "Orthomolecular Medicine." *Journal of the International Academy of Metabology*, vol 5, no. 1, 54–57, 1977.
12. Muramoto, N. *Healing Ourselves*. New York: Avon, 1973.
13. Pearce, J. C. *The Crack in the Cosmic Egg*. New York: Crown, 1976.
14. Cousins, N. "The Holistic Health Revolution." *Saturday Review*, March 31, 1979.
15. Bloomfield, H., *op cit.*
16. Ballentine, R., *op cit.*
17. Muramoto, N., *op cit.*
18. Laszlo, E., *op cit.*

19. Williams, R. J. 1973, *op cit.*
20. Hall, R. H., 1974, *op cit.*
21. Hall, K. "Orthomolecular Therapy: Review of the Literature." *Orthomolecular Psychiatry*, vol 4, no. 4, 297–313, 1975.
22. Hoffer, A. "Treatment of Schizophrenia." *Orthomolecular Psychiatry*, vol. 3, no. 4, 280–290, 1974.
23. Williams, R. J., 1971, *op cit.*
24. Mandell, M. "Cerebral Reactions in Allergic Patients." *Second International Congress of Social Psychiatry, Section on Ecologic Mental Illness,* London, August 8, 1969.
25. Randolph, T. G. "Ecologic Orientation in Medicine. Comprehensive Environmental Control in Diagnosis and Therapy." *Annals of Allergy,* vol. 23, 7–22, 1965.
26. Philpott, W. H. "Maladaptive Reactions to Frequently Used Foods and Commonly Met Chemicals as Precipitating Factors in Many Chronic Physical and Emotional Illnesses." In Williams, R. J. and Kalita, D. K.: *Physicians Handbook of Orthomolecular Medicine,* Elmsford, New York: Pergamon, 1977.
27. Feingold, B. *Why Your Child Is Hyperactive.* New York: Random House, 1975.
28. Feingold, B. "Hyperkinesis and Learning Difficulties." Hearing before the Senate Committee on Nutrition and Human Needs: Diet Related to Killer Diseases, Washington, D.C.: US Govt Printing Office, 1977, page 280.
29. Airola, P. *Hypoglycemia: A Better Approach.* Health Plus, 1977.
30. Fredericks, C. *Low Blood Sugar and You.* New York: Grosset and Dunlap, 1969.
31. Abrahamson, E. M. and Pezet, A. W. *Body, Mind and Sugar.* New York: Holt, Rinehart and Winston, 1951.
32. Cheraskin, Ringsdorf, and Brecher, *Psychodietetics.* Briarcliff Manor, New York: Stein and Day, 1974.
33. Kalita, D. "Hypoglycemia—The End of Your Sweet Life." In Williams et al. *Physicians Handbook on Orthomolecular Medicine.* Elmsford, New York: Pergamon, 1977.
34. Weil, A. *The Natural Mind.* Boston: Houghton Mifflin, 1972.
35. Illich, I. *Medical Nemesis.* New York: Random House, 1976.
36. Muramoto, N., *op cit.*
37. Airola, P. *How to Get Well.* Health Plus, 1974.

The Practice of Holistic Nutrition   pp. 145–57

1. Jacobson, M. *Eater's Digest.* New York: Doubleday, 1974.
2. Hunter, B. T. *Consumer Beware.* New York: Simon and Schuster, 1971.

3. Hunter, B. T. *The Mirage Of Safety.* New York: Scribner's, 1975.

4. Hunter, B. T. *The Great Nutrition Robbery.* New York: Scribner's, 1978.

5. Kindenlehrer, J. *Confessions of a Sneaky Organic Cook.* Emmaus, Pennsylvania: Rodale, 1971.

6. Jensen, B. *The Doctor–Patient Handbook.* Biworld Publications, 1976.

7. Wigmore, A. *Be Your Own Doctor.* New York: Hemisphere, undated.

8. Kulvinskas, V. *Survival into the Twenty-First Century,* Omangod Press, 1975.

9. Ehret, A. *Prof Arnold Ehret's Mucusless Diet Healing System.* Ehret Literature Publishing Co., 1977.

10. Jensen, B., 1976, *op cit.*

11. Kushi, M. "Macrobiotics and Oriental Medicine." *Wholistic Dimensions in Health.* New York: Doubleday, 1978.

12. Hoffer, A. "The Treatment of Schizophrenia," *Journal of Orthomolecular Psychiatry,* vol. 3, no. 4, 280–290, 1974.

13. Feingold, B. *Why Your Child Is Hyperactive.* New York: Random House, 1975.

14. Feingold, B. "Hyperkinesis and Learning Difficulties," Hearing before the Senate Committee on Nutrition and Human Needs: Diet related to Killer Diseases, Washington, D.C.: US Govt Printing Office, 1977, page 280.

15. Airola, P. *How to Get Well.* Health Plus, 1974.

16. Jensen, B., 1976, *op cit.*

17. Jensen, B. *Nature Has a Remedy.* Vanity Publications, 1978.

18. Lappe, F. M. *Diet for a Small Planet.* New York: Ballantine, 1971.

19. Ohsawa, G. *You Are All Sanpaku.* Secaucus, New Jersey: University Books, 1965.

20. Wigmore, A., *op cit.*

21. Gregory, D. "Natural Diet for Folks Who Eat," *Cookin' With Mother Nature.* New York: Harper & Row, 1973.

22. Jensen, B., 1976, *op cit.*

23. Airola, P., 1974, *op cit.*

24. Kulvinskas, V., *op cit.*

25. Wigmore, A., *op cit.*

26. Airola. P., 1974, *op cit.*

27. Ibid.

Beyond Death   pp. 168–76

1. On file at Parastudy, Inc., Valleybrook Road, Chester Heights, Pennsylvania 19017, and conducted by Howell Lewis Shay and Mrs. Evelyn Webber, Spring 1976.

2. Reported from a talk given before the Spiritual Frontiers Fellowship,

November 1970, and based on the speaker's experience at Camp Berkeley, Texas, in 1943. On file at Parastudy, Inc.

3. Moody, Raymond A., Jr., M.D. *Life after Life.* St. Simon's Island, Georgia; Mockingbird Books, 1975.

4. Fuller, John G. *The Ghost of Flight 401,* and *The Airmen Who Would Not Die.* New York: Putnam, 1976, 1979.

5. Greaves, Helen. "Testimony of Light." *Churches' Fellowship for Psychical and Spiritual Studies.* London, 1969.

6. Based on the author's experience.

Meditation: A New Way of Being   pp. 190–92

1. LeShan, Lawrence. *How to Meditate: A Guide to Self-Discovery.* Boston: Little, Brown, 1974.

Clearing Negative Influences from the Mind   pp. 234–41

1. Tart, Charles T., ed. *Altered States of Consciousness.* New York: Doubleday (Anchor), 1972.

2. Selye, Hans, M.D. *The Stress of Life.* New York: McGraw-Hill, 1976.

3. Kübler-Ross, Elizabeth. *Death.* Englewood Cliffs, New Jersey: Prentice-Hall, 1975.

4. Wickland, Carl A., M.D. *Thirty Years among the Dead.* North Hollywood, California: Newcastle Publishing Co., 1924. (Recently reprinted.)

5. Selye, *op cit.*

6. Finch, William J. *The Pendulum and Possession* (revised edition). Sedona, Arizona: Esoteric Publications, 1975.

7. Neville. *Resurrection.* Marina del Rey, California: D. E. Vorss & Co., 1966.

8. Finch, *op cit.*

9. Lilly, John C. *Programming and Metaprogramming in the Human Biocomputer.* New York: Julian Press, 1967, 1972.

A Bird's-Eye View of Oriental Medicine   pp. 249–62

1. *See* Tohei, K. *Book of Ki: Coordinating Mind and Body in Daily Life.* New York: Japan Publications, 1976.

2. *See,* for example, Carlson, R. *The Frontiers of Science and Medicine.* South Bend, Indiana: Regnery/Gateway, 1975, pp. 180–219.

3. *See* Kushi, M. *The Macrobiotic Way of Natural Healing.* Boston: East-West Publications, 1978, pp. 34–75.

The Longest Stride of Soul Man Ever Took   pp. 285–92

1. Bucke, Richard. *Cosmic Consciousness.* New York: Universe, 1961.
2. Bailey, Alice A. *The Rays & the Initiations.* New York: Lucius, 1972.
3. Ibid.

Selected Reading

Biofeedback

Butler, Francine. *Biofeedback—A Survey of the Literature.* New York: IFl/Plenum Data Co., 1974.

Brown, Barbara. *New Mind, New Body.* New York: Harper and Row, 1974.

———. *Stress and the Art of Biofeedback.* New York: Harper and Row, 1977.

Cade, C. Maxwell, and Nona Coxhead. *The Awakened Mind.* New York: Delacorte, 1979.

Green, Elmer, and Alyce Green. *Beyond Biofeedback.* New York: Dell, 1977.

Birth and Before

Annas, Geroge. *The Rights of Hospital Patients.* New York: Avon, 1976.

Banat, Barbara, and Mary L. Rodzilsky. *What Now?* New York: Scribner's, 1975.

Bean, Constance. *Methods of Childbirth.* New York: Doubleday, 1974.

Boston Women's Health Book Collective. *Ourselves and Our Children.* New York: Random House, 1978.

Brewer, Gail S. *The Pregnancy After 30 Workbook.* Emmaus, Pa.: Rodale, 1978.

———. *What Every Pregnant Woman Should Know—The Truth About Diet and Drugs in Pregnancy.* New York: Random House, 1977.

Chabon, Irwin. *Awake and Aware.* New York: Delacorte, 1969.

Donovan, Bonnie. *The Cesarian Birth Experience.* Boston: Beacon, 1978.

Ewy, Donna and Rodger. *Preparation for Breastfeeding.* New York: Doubleday, 1975.

———. *Preparation for Childbirth.* New York: Signet–New American Library, 1974.

Hazell, Lester D. *Commonsense Childbirth.* New York: Berkley, 1976.

Karmel, Marjorie. *Thank You Dr. Lamaze.* New York: Doubleday, 1959.

Leboyer, Frederick. *Birth Without Violence.* New York: Knopf, 1975.

Noble, Elizabeth. *Essential Exercises for the Childbearing Year.* Boston: Houghton Mifflin, 1976.

312

Shneour, Elie. *The Malnourished Mind*. New York: Doubleday, 1974.

Sousa, Marion. *Childbirth at Home*. New York: Bantam, 1976.

Williams, Phyllis. *Nourishing Your Unborn Child*. New York: Avon, 1975.

Cancer

Gerson, Max. *A Cancer Therapy*. Del Mar, Cal.: Totality Books, 1958.

Hutschnecker, Arnold A. *The Will to Live*. New York: Simon and Schuster, 1974.

Simonton, O. Carl; Stephanie Matthews-Simonton; James Creighton. *Getting Well Again*. Los Angeles: J. P. Tarcher, 1978.

Death, Dying and Beyond

Becker, Ernest. *The Denial of Death*. New York: Macmillan, 1973.

Dunne, John S. *The City of the Gods*. Notre Dame, Ind.: University of Notre Dame, 1965.

Fuller, John G. *The Ghost of Flight 401*. New York: Berkley, 1976.

Grof, Stanislav and Joan Halifax. *The Human Encounter with Death*. New York: E. P. Dutton, 1977.

Grollman, Earl A. *Talking About Death*. Boston: Beacon, 1976.

Kavanaugh, Robert E. *Facing Death*. New York: Penguin, 1972.

Kübler-Ross, Elisabeth. *On Death and Dying*. New York: Macmillan, 1969.

———. *Death: The Final Stage of Growth*. Englewood Cliffs, N.J.: Prentice-Hall, 1975.

Lee, Laurel. *Walking Through The Fire*. New York: Bantam, 1977.

Levine, Stephen. *A Gradual Awakening*. Garden City, N.Y.: Doubleday, 1979.

Moody, Raymond A. Jr. *Life After Life*. New York: Bantam, 1975.

Diet and Nutrition

Abrahamson, E. M. and A. W. Pezet. *Body, Mind and Sugar*. New York: Holt, Rinehart and Winston, 1951.

Airola, Paavo. *How to Get Well*. Phoenix: Health Plus, 1974.

———. *How To Keep Slim, Healthy and Young with Juice Fasting*. Phoenix: Health Plus, 1971.

———. *Hypoglycemia*. Phoenix: Health Plus, 1977.

Albright, Nancy. *The Rodale Cookbook*. Emmaus, Pa.: Rodale, 1973.

Ballentine, Rudolph, M.D. *Diet and Nutrition.* Honesdale, Pa.: The Himalayan International Institute, 1978.

Cheraskin, E.; W. M. Ringsdorf, Jr.; Arline Brecher. *Psychodietetics.* New York: Bantam, 1976.

Davis, Adele. *Let's Cook It Right.* New York: Harcourt Brace Jovanovich, 1962.

Dworkin, S. and F. *Bend It Splendid.* Emmaus, Pa.: Rodale, 1973.

―――. *The Good Goodies.* Emmaus, Pa.: Rodale, 1974.

Ewald, E. B. *Recipes for a Small Planet.* New York: Ballantine, 1973.

Ford, Marjorie W.; Susan Hillyard; Mary Faulk Koock. *The Deaf Smith Cookbook.* New York: Macmillan―Collier, 1973.

Friedlander, B. *The Findhorn Cookbook.* New York: Grosset and Dunlap, 1976.

Goldbeck, N. and D. *The Supermarket Handbook.* New York: Signet, 1974.

Gregory, Dick. *Natural Diet for Folks Who Eat; Cookin' with Mother Nature.* New York: Harper and Row, 1973.

Hall, Ross Hume. *Food for Nought: The Decline in Nutrition.* New York: Vintage, 1976.

Hunter, B. T. *The Natural Foods Cookbook.* New York: Pyramid, 1967.

―――. *The Natural Foods Primer.* New York: Simon and Schuster, 1972.

Jensen, Bernard. *Nature Has a Remedy.* Atlanta: Vanity Publishers, 1978.

―――. *The Doctor Patient Handbook.* Provo, Utah: Biworld Publications, 1976.

Katzen, M. *The Moosewood Cookbook.* Berkeley, Cal.: Ten Speed, 1977.

Keyes, Elizabeth and Paul K. Chivington. *What's Eating You?* Marina del Rey, Cal.: DeVorss, 1978.

Kulvinskas, Viktoras. *The Survival into the Twenty-First Century.* California: Omangod, 1975.

Kushi, Michio. "Macro-biotics and Oriental Medicine." In Kaslof, L., ed., *Dimensions in Healing.* New York: Doubleday, 1978.

Lappe, Frances Moore. *Diet for a Small Planet.* New York: Ballantine, 1971.

McCausland, Marcus. *Nutrition Research: The Need for an Innovative Approach.* 1 A Addison Crescent, London, England: Privately printed by Marcus McCausland.

Muramoto, Naboru. *Healing Ourselves.* New York: Avon, 1973.

Otisawa, Georges. *You Are All Sanpaku.* New Jersey: University Books, 1965.

Peshek, Robert J. D.D.S. *Balancing Body Chemistry with Nutrition.* Riverside, Cal.: Color Coded Systems Publishers, 1977.

Robertson, L.; C. Flinders; G. Bronwen. *Laurel's Kitchen.* Petaluma, Cal.: Nilgiri Press, 1976.

Thomas, Anna. *The Vegetarian Epicure.* New York: Vintage, 1972.

Watson, George. *Nutrition and Your Mind.* New York: Harper and Row, 1972.

Williams, Roger J. *Biochemical Individuality.* Austin, Texas: Univ. of Texas Press, 1956.

Williams, R. *Nutrition Against Disease.* New York: Pitman, 1971.

Exercise and the Physical Body

Barlow, Wilfred. *The Alexander Technique.* New York: Alfred A. Knopf, 1977.

Cooper, Kenneth. *The New Aerobics.* New York: Bantam, 1970.

General

Bentov, Itzhak. *Stalking the Wild Pendulum.* New York: Bantam, 1977.

Capra, Fritjof. *The Tao of Physics.* New York: Bantam, 1977.

Findhorn Community. *The Findhorn Garden.* New York: Harper and Row, 1968.

Harper, Kate. *The Childfree Alternative.* Brattleboro, Vt.: The Stephen Greene Press, 1980.

Illich, Ivan. *Medical Nemesis: The Expropriation of Health.* New York: Random House, 1976.

Leonard, George. *The Silent Pulse.* New York: E. P. Dutton, 1978.

Michell, John. *The View Over Atlantis.* New York: Ballantine, 1969.

Ostrander, Sheila, and Lynn Schroeder. *Psychic Discoveries Behind the Iron Curtain.* New York: Bantam, 1971.

Page, Irvine H. "Science, Intuition and Medical Practice". *Postgraduate Medicine* 64: 217–221.

Panati, Charles. *Supersenses.* Garden City, N.Y.: Anchor, 1976.

Pearce, Joseph Chilton. *The Crack in the Cosmic Egg.* New York: Pocket, 1976.

Selye, Hans. *Stress without Distress.* Philadelphia: J. B. Lippincott, 1974.

Tompkins, Peter, and Christopher Bird. *The Secret Life of Planets.* New York: Avon, 1973.

Watson, Lyall. *Supernature.* London, England: Hodder and Stoughton, 1973.

Weed, Lawrence L. *Your Health Care and How to Manage It.* Burlington, Vt.: PROMIS Laboratory, University of Vermont, 1975.

Weil, A. *The Natural Mind.* Boston: Houghton-Mifflin, 1972.

Herbs and Herbal Medicine

Bethel, May. *The Healing Power of Herbs.* No. Hollywood, Cal.: Wilshire Book Co., 1977.

Dawson, Adele G. *Health, Happiness and the Pursuit of Herbs.* Brattleboro, Vt.: The Stephen Greene Press, 1980.

Gosling, Nalda. *Herbs for Colds and Flu.* England: Thorsons Publishers Ltd., 1976.

Kloss, Jethro. *Back to Eden.* Santa Barbara, Cal.: Woodbridge, 1939.

Lust, John. *The Herb Book.* New York: Bantam, 1974.

Medsger, Oliver Perry. *Edible Wild Plants.* New York: Collier-Macmillan, 1966.

Meyer, Joseph E. *The Herbalist.* Glenwood, Ill.: Meyerbooks, 1918.

Szekely, Edmond Bordeaux. *The Book of Herbs.* Costa Rica: International Biogenic Society, 1978.

Thomson, William A. R. *Herbs That Heal.* New York: Scribners, 1976.

Holistic Health

Ardell, Donald B. "High Level Wellness and the HSAs: A Health Planning Success Story." *American Journal of Health Planning.* 3: 1–18.

Barny, Helen L., and Louis M. Savary. *Music and Your Mind: Listening with a New Consciousness.* New York: Harper and Row, 1973.

Cousins, Norman. "What I Learned from 3,000 Doctors." *Saturday Review* (Feb. 18, 1978): 12–16.

Forbes, Alec. *Try Being Healthy.* Plymouth, England: Langdon, 1976.

Fordyce, Wilbert E. *Behavioral Methods for Chronic Pain and Illness.* St. Louis, Mo.: C. V. Mosby, 1976.

Frank, Jerome D. "The Medical Power of Faith." *Human Nature* (August, 1978): 40–47.

Grace, William J., et al. "Graduated Patient Responsibility." *Journal of the American Medical Association* 231: 351.

Halpern, Steven. *Spectrum Suite.* Palo Alto, Cal.: SRI Records and Tapens, 1976.

Hill, Ann, Ed. *A Visual Encyclopedia of Unconventional Medicine.* New York: Crown, 1979.

Kaslof, Leslie J. *Wholistic Dimensions in Healing.* Garden City, N.Y.: Doubleday, 1972.

Loomis, Ewarts G., and J. Sig Paulson. *Healing for Everyone: Medicine of the Whole Person.* New York: Hawthorne, 1975.

Menninger, Roy W. "Psychiatry 1976: Time for a Holistic Medicine." *Annals of Internal Medicine* 84: 603–604.

Osler, Sir William. *The Principles and Practice of Medicine.* Chicago: Daniel Appleton, 1912.

Schultz, Johannes, and Wolfgang Luthe. *Autogenic Therapy.* New York: Grune and Stratton, 1969.

Shealy, C. Norman. *Biogenic Health Maintenance.* LaCrosse, Wisconsin: Self-Health Systems, 1976.

————. "Electrical Stimulation of Skin, Peripheral Nerves, and Spinal Dorsal Columns for Control of Pain: A 6½ Year Experience." *Handbook of Medical Acupunture.* New York: Van Nostrand Reinhold, 1976.

————. *The Pain Game.* Millbrae, Cal.: Celestial Arts, 1976.

Soyka, Fred and Alan Edmonds. *The Ion Effect.* New York: Bantam, 1978.

Williams, R. J., and D. K. Kalita. *A Physician's Handbook on Orthomolecular Medicine.* New York: Pergamon, 1977.

Kinesiology

Diamond, John. *Behavioral Kinesiology.* New York: Harper and Row, 1979.

Goodheart, George J. *Applied Kinesiology: 1976 Workshop Procedure Manual.* Detroit, Mich.: 1976.

Stoner, Fred. *The Eclectic Approach to Chiropractic.* Las Vegas, Nev.: F.L.S., 1976.

Thie, John F., ed. Collected Papers of the Diplomates of the International College of Applied Kinesiology. Los Angeles: T. H. Enterprises, 1977.

Thie, John F., with Mary Marks. *Touch For Health.* Santa Monica, Cal.: DeVorss, 1973.

Walther, David D. *Applied Kinesiology: The Advanced Approach in Chiropractic.* Pueblo, Colo.: Systems, DC, 1976.

Meditation and Relaxation

Benson, Herbert. *The Relaxation Response.* New York: Morrow, 1975.

Davis, Roy Eugene. *An Easy Guide to Meditation.* Lakemont, Ga.: CSA, 1978.

Forem, Jack. *Transcendental Meditation.* New York: E. P. Dutton, 1973.

Jacobson, Edmund. *Progressive Relaxation.* Chicago: University of Chicago, 1929.

Kanellakos, D. P., and J. P. Lucas. *The Psychobiology of Transcendental Meditation.* Hunter, N.Y.: W. A. Benjamin, 1974.

Khan, Pir Vilayat Inayat, and George Trevelyan. *New Age Meditations.* London: Winged Heart, 1971.

LeShan, Lawrence. *How to Meditate.* Boston: Little Brown, 1974.

Mandelkom, Philip, ed. *To Know Yourself.* Garden City, N.Y.: 1978.

Merton, Thomas. *New Seeds of Contemplation.* New York: New Directions, 1961.

Oyle, Irving. *The Healing Mind.* New York: Pocket, 1976.

Prabhavananda, Swami, and Christopher Isherwood. *How to Know God: The Yoga Aphorisms of Patanjali.* Hollywood, Cal.: Vedanta, 1971.

Satchidananda, Swami Sri. *Meditation.* New York: Integral Yoga Institute, 1972.

Sivananda, Swami. *Concentration and Meditation.* Durban, South Africa: Divine Life Society, 1965.

Stearn, Jess. *The Power of Alpha Thinking.* New York: Signet—New American Library, 1977.

Mind and Brain

Ferguson, Marilyn. *The Brain Revolution.* New York: Bantam, 1975.

Finch, Elizabeth and Bill. *The Pendulum and Your Health.* Sedona, Ariz.: Esoteric Publications, 1977.

Pelletier, Kenneth. *Mind as Healer, Mind as Slayer.* New York: Delacorte, 1977.

Oriental Medicine

Bendix, G. *Press Point Therapy.* New York: Avon, 1978.

Lawson-Wood, D. and J. *Acupuncture Handbook.* Sussex, England: Health Science Press, 1973.

McGarey, William A. *Acupuncture and Body Energies.* Phoenix, Ariz.: Gabriel. 1974.

Wett, George. "Acupuncture: Pricking the Bubble of Skepticism." In *Biological Psychiatry* 13: 159–161.

Psychic Healing

Boyd, Doug. *Rolling Thunder*. New York: Dell, 1974.

Hoffman, Enid. *Huna: A Beginners' Guide*. Gloucester, Mass.: Para Research, 1976.

Karagulla, Shafica. *Breakthrough to Creativity*. Santa Monica, Cal.: DeVorss, 1967.

Psychology

Assagioli, Roberto. *Psychosynthesis*. New York: Viking, 1971.

Coue, Emile, and C. H. Brooks. *Suggestion and Autosuggestion*. New York: Samuel Weiser, 1974.

Harris, Thomas A. *I'm OK—You're OK*. New York: Harper and Row, 1967.

Remen, Naomi. *The Masculine Principle, the Feminine Principle and Humanistic Medicine*. San Francisco, Cal.: Institute for the Study of Humanistic Medicine, 1975.

Reflexology/Prenatal Therapy

Berkson, Devaki. *The Footbook*. New York: Funk and Wagnalls, 1977.

Carter, Mildred. *Helping Yourself with Foot Reflexology*. West Nyack, N.Y.: Parker, 1969.

Ingham, Eunice D. *Stories the Feet Can Tell, Stories the Feet Have Told*. Rochester, N.Y.: Eunice D. Ingham, 1951.

St. John, Robert. *Metamorphosis*. 17 Berewecke Road, Winchester, England: Printed and published by Robert St. John, 1976.

————. *Prenatal Therapy*. (Pamphlet) Winchester, England: Robert St. John, no date.

Relationships

Jackins, Harvey. *The Human Side of Human Beings*. Seattle: Rational Island, 1965.

————. *The Upward Trend*. Seattle: Rational Island, 1977.

Satir, Virginia. *Peoplemaking*. Palo Alto, Cal.: Science and Behavior, 1972.

Sexuality

Boston Women's Health Collective. *Our Bodies, Ourselves*. New York: Simon and Schuster, 1973.

Morrison, Eleanor S., and Mila Underhill Price. *Values in Sexuality: A New Approach to Sex Education.* New York: Hart, 1974.

Nofziger, Margaret. *A Cooperative Method of Natural Birth Control.* Summertown, Tenn.: The Book Publishing Co., 1976.

Silbergeld, Bernie. *Male Sexuality.* Boston: Little Brown, 1978.

Spirituality

Bailey, Alice A. *Esoteric Healing.* New York and London: Lucis, 1953.

———. *Treatise on White Magic.* New York and London: Lucis, 1971.

Bucke, Richard. *Cosmic Consciousness.* New York: Universe, 1961.

Solomon, Paul. *The Paul Solomon Tapes.* Virginia Beach, Va.: Fellowship of the Inner Light, 1974.

Szekely, Edmond Bordeaux. *The Essene Way Biogenic Living.* Costa Rica: International Biogenic Society, 1978.

Index

Medical schools, 27, 52
Meditation, 17-8, 53, 58, 60, 108, 190-2, 193-7
transcendental, 46, 190
Menninger Clinic, 46
Menninger Foundation, 208, 213
Mental retardation, 140
Miller, Neal, 205
Moody, Raymond A., Jr., 169, 171
Moses, 5-6
Mullholland, Joseph, 205
Muramoto, N., 143

Nanikoshi, Tokujiro, 225
National Cancer Institute, 59
National Health Service, 272, 277
National Institutes of Health, 59
National Organization for Optional Parenthood, 78
Native Americans, 48
Neanderthal man, 198
Neurosis, 140
New England Journal of Medicine, 60
Nitrogen mustard, 60
Noyes, Russell, 169

Ohsawa, Georges, 156
Oriental Five-Element Theory, 136
Oriental medicine, 46, 136, 143
Osis, Karlis, 169, 170-1
Ott, John N., 120

Parapsychology Foundation, 172
Pasteur, Louis, 49
Pearce, Ian, 56, 60-1
Pellagra, 132
Peshek, Robert, 247
Petroleum industry, 50
Pharmacology, 50
Physicians, 24, 26, 28, 29, 31, 47, 83, 85, 86-7, 108, 189, 279
Poliomyelitis, 53
Pregnancy, 83-9
Prenatal therapy, 225-33
Principles of Medical Ethics, 47
Proverbs, Book of, 5-6
Psychic Power of Running, 118
Psychical Research Foundation, 171
Psychosomatic medicine, 4-6 *passim*

Raab, W., 114
Radiesthesia, 36
Radionics, 46
Rama, Swami, 191, 213
Rays and Initiations, 286
Recommended Daily Allowances, 133, 140

Reflexology, 46
Rockwell, Norman, 126
Roentgen, W. K., 49

St. Gall, 203
St. John, Robert, 227-32
St. Pierre, 232-3
San Andreas Yoga Center, 119
Sanger, Margaret, 73
Samadhi, 196, 213
Schultz, Johannes, 213
Scurvy, 132
Self-healing, 37-9, 216-24
Selye, Hans, 207
Sepulveda Veterans' Hospital, 205
Sex education, 73-5
Sexuality, 71-80
Sheehan, George, 111
Shock, H., 114
Silent Pulse, The, 233
Silva Mind Control, 190
Simonton, O. Carl, 56, 60, 109, 187
Simonton, Stephanie, 187
Smallpox, 49, 53
Smuts, Jan Christian, ix
Specialists, specialization, 3, 23, 31, 51
Spirit, 122-5, 136
Standard American Diet, 145, 153, 156
Stanford Research Institute, 171
Stimulation, 187-8
Stravinsky, Igor, 34-5
Stress, 112-3, 207-8, 237-8
Stoffels, Herbert, 247
Sympto-thermal method. *See* birth control
Synergism, 7
Synergistic healing, 5
Szekely, Edmond Bordeaux, 128

T'ai Chi, 250, 252, 261
TEMP, 205, 208
Therapeutae, 16
Triune concept, 3

Ultra-sensing, 174-5
University of California, 171
University of Dublin, 172
University of Iowa College of Medicine, 169
University of Toronto, 114
University of Virginia Medical School, 171

Vibration, 183-4, 185-6
Visual imagery, 60
Vitamins, 132, 139-40, 144, 153

Date Due

SEP 24 '93			
OCT 1 3 '93			
MAY 3 1 1999			